MASCARA BOY

MASCARA BOY

BULLIED, ASSAULTED, & NEAR DEATH: **SURVIVING TRAUMA & ADDICTION**

BRANDON LEE

First paperback edition June 2019

Edited by John Peragine
Cover Art by Brandon Lee

978-1-7338587-0-0 (Hardback)
978-1-7338587-1-7 (Paperback)

Published by Rock Bottom Media

Acknowledgement

I want to thank my recovery sponsor, CeCe, for guiding me through the 12 Steps and encouraging me to love myself the way others love me. A special shout out to my sister Stephanie who, no matter what, loves and supports my mission to help save the lives of addicts who are suffering. Thanks to my best friend, Tyler, who kept encouraging me to put pen to paper knowing that my story can help others even when I doubted myself. Thank you to my editor, John, who really helped me find the right words to express my message, and for helping me create the title of the book, *Mascara Boy*.

Lastly, I want to thank my higher power and the 12 Step Recovery Program of which I am a current member. You've all given me the strength to write down some of my most painful memories so that others can find hope despite addiction.

This book is dedicated to the 23 million Americans who are addicted to drugs and alcohol. It's also for those friends and family members of addicts who feel helpless and hopeless while watching their loved ones suffer. This book is for all of you. This book is about my experience, strength, and hope so that you can create the life you never thought possible.

Table of Contents

Introduction

The stain of addiction threatens my livelihood. I have so much to lose, so why am I doing this? I am doing it for you, my readers. If I have to fall on the proverbial sword in order to get rid of the stigma of addiction for those in recovery, and those who love someone in recovery, then it is worth every possible missed opportunity. Recovery saves lives -in the literal sense, and in the sense that those who survive have a life they can rebuild.

We are labeled as "trouble" and "dangerous." In the professional world we are labeled as "high-risk hires." I challenge the thinking of every boss who owns a small business to corporate CEOs of large media conglomerates. I am living proof that your judgements are misguided and created out of fear.

Addicts who are living in their active disease can very well be dangerous. It is imperative that we give each and every one of them the opportunity at a new life. There is no one who is truly lost, only those who have not found their way yet.

Addicts in active recovery, on the other hand, can prove to be some of the most honest, truthful, dedicated, loyal employees in the workforce. As an addict who works the 12 Steps every second of every day of my life, I can tell you that I do everything I can to NOT lie, steal, cheat. I am accountable to my higher power, my God, and I confess all of my wrong-doings and promise to make amends, or simply put, to make it right.

Here's something you should know: addicts do everything we can to NOT have to make amends. It is uncomfortable, and so we try to avoid making the mistake to begin with. We try our best to be authentic, truthful, and honest because we have seen what happens when we lose sight of our moral compass. And we work on bettering our lives every day.

Why would I risk everything by coming out of the multi-room closet and confess to the world who I was, who I am, and who I hope to become? It has been a high-risk gamble. I have had two major job offers rescinded because executives made a snap judgment about my past, instead of taking the time to get to know the man I am today.

I don't profess to understand the workings of someone else's mind or personal values, but I can make an educated guess based upon my own experiences, and of those whom I have met on my journey. When someone hears you had trouble in the past with drugs, they look at you as some foul-smelling stain coalesces in their minds. *Once an addict, always an addict. It is just a matter of time before they use again, because an addict is essentially a flawed human being.*

If we have learned anything about the opioid crisis, it is that addiction is an opportunistic disease, one that does not discriminate based upon race, creed, religion, marital status, whether you are a parent, whether you are a Sunday school teacher or CEO of a Fortune 500 company. It can grip an unwary victim, dig its claws deep into a person, and wreck their lives. But does that mean we should give up on that person?

Was it ever an option for the people of New Orleans to throw up their hands, say their city was lost forever, and just walk away? Hurricane Katrina was a terrible, destructive tragedy, but people came back and rebuilt the city better than it was previously.

I was working in New York City and living near Ground Zero on 9/11. It took me many years to return to that spot, but the memorials and structures there, while a reminder of the past, in no way make the statement of giving up. New Yorkers never give up on anything. We rebuilt bigger, better, and more badass.

The life of an active addict is destructive and it can take down the lives of those around them, but once the storm has passed and the rebuilding has taken place, why do people choose to only see the tragedy rather than the whole person standing before them? I admit I don't have an answer to that, but that should never discourage an addict from getting help and creating a bright future—haters be damned!

There is a growing issue in America. We stigmatize an entire group of people as bad. We marginalize them and act as though they are disposable. We label people as trash and distance ourselves from them, as if befriending them will expose us to some sort of social disease.

Because of this prevalent mindset, many recovering addicts fear telling people about their past struggles because they fear others will judge them harshly. Maybe they'll be denied a promotion for sharing their story or denied a potential position. There may be some truth, as I have experienced this type of discrimination, but I am still standing. I am still strong. I am pushing forward every day toward new goals, and I am achieving new heights. The crap exists, but I choose to not let it define my life.

Every one of us has done something shameful in our lives. We ALL have skeletons in the closet. The people who lock those skeletons in the closet and throw away the key often feel threatened by others who are brave enough to rip the skeletons out of the closet and into the open. They fear being exposed themselves. They become nervous about people finding out about their past.

You will read about this prison cell that I kept next to my heart for too many years. I was so worried I would not be able to handle the emotions and experiences that I had buried there. Eventually the door was blown down, and I dealt with the demons that existed there. Once I did, I became whole for the first time in my life.

Many people fear that room in their heart, fear that letting out the demons will consume them. The truth is we don't have to do it alone. There is help and where there is help, there is hope.

When people keep those inner demons, those secrets, those shameful memories locked away, they become fearful, and that fear, turned outward, can become hate. Hate born out of self-loathing. The more they see others brave enough to become free, the more they feel ashamed that they cannot, or more accurately, will not, deal with their own issues and past.

I cannot change others. I cannot be responsible for others' issues. Those people who choose to shame me or judge me for my past don't deserve me at my present.

I am here to share my story publicly because I hope that stepping forward, sharing my full name and showing my face, and not hiding in anonymity, will remove some of the stigma of recovering addicts and open the hearts and minds of older generations. I hope to one day jump back into a chaotic newsroom covering stories that impact our community. But, if writing this book never allows that to happen, it's a risk that I am willing to take, because as I always say: what the hell was the point of suffering all that pain if that pain can't help someone else live a better life.

1

Sex Abuse Issues

O ne of the reasons I was inspired to write my story and share it with the world is that many people like me are suffering. It is my sincerest hope that you are reading this book sometime in the future and seeing the world I am currently living in as some dark blip in history. A smear that was dark and oily but which has been cleaned up and relegated to the history books as a warning that no human being should ever endure sex abuse shame. I am under no illusion that sex abuse will vanish from society forever, as we will always have twisted individuals born into our world with horrific agendas and thirsts for acts that belong in the lowest levels of hell.

The dark oily stain that lies upon our current society is one made up of complacency and denial, and one in which victims are seen as deserving of further victimization. As if their lives are not already derailed, they are now a target for disdain, mockery, and humiliation.

Why would any sane person disclose sexual abuse in the current climate in which I am writing this book? I use the word "sane," because I must consider the consequences of such a disclosure. Either the person is so traumatized that they disclose in order to finally unburden their shredded soul, or if they are making up a story of abuse they still must be someone in pain and have some serious mental health issues. The fallout is just too great for someone to come forward because they risk losing everything in the process—their family, their career, their status in their community, their status among their peers—when the shame that they have carried for years is revealed on the public stage. A person who claims to be a victim must be prepared to be ridiculed and ostracized. There is no possible motive for gain, as justice for such disclosures has become nothing but a punchline for most victims. Not all victims, but most.

PIANO LESSONS

When I was a boy, my parents wanted us kids to be well-rounded. I played baseball, basketball, soccer, and tennis. My parents also believed we should learn to play music. When I was about 10 years old I decided to play piano, and my parents found a teacher. We had one of those big grand pianos in the living room that almost looked too pretty to touch. I was excited for my first lesson. The teacher came to our house in the late afternoon after I got home from school. He came once a week.

I sat on the piano bench and my teacher sat next to me, side by side. He began teaching me the basics, but as a young boy I made lots of mistakes. I will never forget that first mistake. I messed up the very simple "do.. re.. mi .. fa .. so.." That's when it happened. He touched me. I had never been touched like that before. My body cringed and then I froze. I tried not to mess up. I started playing again. Sure enough, I hit the wrong key. My body tensed up. I knew something was going to happen. My teacher groped me again.

He eventually left that day. My first piano lesson was over. A full week went by. I didn't say anything. I acted as if nothing happened and nothing was wrong. I put a smile on my face, but inside I was hurting.

The following Friday, I started to shiver. It was lesson time again. I knew the teacher was coming over. I ran straight into my room and jumped into my bed under the covers. I even remember using pillows to build a little fort, thinking that I would be safe. When my mom told me it was time for my lesson, I told her, "Mom, I don't feel good. I can't play the piano today."

Everyone brushed it off as me being a typical kid, just being difficult. He came into the room and pulled off the pillows one by one until I was exposed and I had no choice but to go to the living room and sit at the piano. I remember that scene so vividly. I slowly walked to the bench with my head down. To the outward observer, I looked like a kid who was pouting. I sat down and started to play. I kept telling myself, "Don't mess up. Don't mess up. Don't mess up!" I messed up.

If I hit the wrong key, he would stick his tongue in my ear. The next mistake, he would bite my ear. The next mistake, he would grope me in my private area. The touching got worse and more graphic. I was terrified of the man, and my mother became more annoyed with me the more I tried to refuse to see him.

It would be another 30 years before I confronted my mother about what happened.

Why is there a statute of limitations on sexual assault? It can take years of soul healing and therapy before someone is in a stable enough place to take a perpetrator on in court. Unfortunately, if there was any physical evidence, it is long gone, and those who might know something often just want to turn their heads and leave well enough alone.

It takes time- sometimes years to deal with trauma. The victim often suppresses the memories and feelings deep within themselves. They do this as a coping mechanism, a way to survive. The mind will protect us from trauma the best way it can, and sometimes it does this by suppressing our memories and blurring the details.

A victim of sexual assault is a survivor. It is not just about the initial trauma, it is about the echoes of that trauma that make them relive the event every day. Victims often develop post traumatic stress disorder (PTSD) similar to what soldiers experience when they return from the battlefield. They experience this loop in time in which they relive the event, over and over. The mind copes by trying to suppress this, because the hurt is so deep it can lead to suicide if untreated.

Some victims are more successful than others. Some get help before it consumes their lives. Others are not as lucky. They self-medicate. They hurt their bodies. They destroy relationships. Their health suffers. They might become obese in order to be less attractive. They may stop bathing. Stop caring about their appearance. They may just stop caring about anything.

BOOM BOOM ROOM

When I was young, my family moved to Corona Del Mar, a quiet little beach town sandwiched between Newport Beach and Laguna Beach. I call it the 8th World Wonder. It's that beautiful.

I often refer to my time attending Catholic high school by comparing it to the pop culture movie *Cruel Intentions* starring Ryan Phillippe and Sarah Michelle Geller. The movie is about really rich Catholic school kids who get wasted on cocaine in high school and play evil tricks on other students. The school I went to was filled with rich kids. Most of our parents worked tirelessly around the clock. Many parents were entrepreneurs. Some kids even got front-row parking with their name on it because mommy and daddy paid for it by donating the most money to the school. Because most of our parents were successful meant they often weren't around because they were working. Most of my friends rarely saw our parents during the school week. It was the norm for our parents to give us cash or let us grab unlimited amounts of cash from the house.

My first experience with hard-core drugs happened when I was about 15. One of my friends bought cocaine and brought it to a friend's beach house. It was his family's vacation home, which meant there were no parents and no supervision. We did lines of cocaine on the coffee table, blaring rap and hip hop music, while staring out into the ocean. Not a bad life at the time for a bunch of teens, right? While we all got wasted, that's when my double life began.

During the late 80s early 90s, Laguna Beach was the epicenter of the gay world. West Hollywood wasn't like what it is today, lined with gay bars and nightclubs. Laguna Beach had two gay bars and a hotel. The most popular back in the day was a place called the Boom Boom Room. I know--I laugh too every time I tell someone about it. There was a lot of "Boom Boom" that happened at this rundown hotel with million-dollar views. The hotel was upstairs. The bar and club were on the first floor. As a very young teen, I used my oldest sister's boyfriend's ID to get into the bars. Back then, no one ever really checked IDs in Laguna, especially at the gay bars. I had it just in case.

One night I was high on drugs. My friends were wasted and hooking up with girls we had met at the beach that day. I decided to sneak away and walk about two miles down the road to the Boom Boom Room. I remember having butterflies in my stomach. Hormones raging. Adrenaline pumping. I had never been inside a gay bar. I had never even kissed a guy before.

I walked straight into the bar and it was sensory overload. The bartenders were shirtless. Their muscles bulged as if they had just finished a pump at the gym. They were like gods to me. I ordered a drink and sat there at the bar gazing at all the gay men around me.

Eventually I wandered outside and noticed guys coming and going from a staircase at the end of the block down to the beach. Curious, I walked over to the staircase. I noticed guys checking me out. No one was talking to each other. Each guy stood a few feet apart from the others, but again, they weren't chatting. Instead they were checking out the steady stream of guys coming up and down the staircase. I could hear the ocean waves crashing, but it was so dark you couldn't see the water. Heck, I couldn't even see the bottom of the winding staircase. Because I was wasted my next move seemed logical; I had to go down.

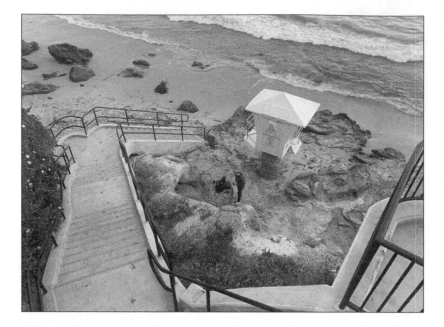

I started winding down the staircase and felt the touch of a man's hand as I passed. One guy touched my chest and whispered something to me. A few feet away I felt another man graze my ass. I was nervous and scared, but I kept going all the way down. That's when a guy grabbed me and pulled me toward him. He began kissing me. Even though I was about 15 at the time, the guys who were cruising the beach were around 40 to 60 years old. I would return to this winding staircase countless times. Each time, the sexual encounters progressed far beyond just kissing.

When I was a kid, I was always shown by society how life was supposed to work. Grow up. Fall in love with a woman. Get married. Have children. Raise a family, and so on. There was a societal structure to follow. Now, imagine life as a gay kid in the 80s and 90s when we were taught that gay people were dying of AIDS as a form of punishment by God. Being gay was a one-way ticket to hell. Gay sex was a sin! Here's the most ridiculous thing I was taught in Catholic school: You can be gay, you just can't have gay sex. I mean, how ridiculous is that? Unless, of course, you're clergy, and then anything goes.

As a gay kid, I had no societal structure to follow. I was told I was going to burn in hell. I could never get married. I could never have or raise children. As a gay man, certain segments of society think I'm a pervert who wants to have sex with children. This is what gays kids heard over and over again growing up in America during that time. So, tell me again why anyone would be shocked when a gay teen at 15 would seek a life of escape by getting wasted on drugs and having sex with much older men at the beach. No one should be shocked. It's actually quite simple to understand.

I never was given hope that I could get married or raise a family. Instead, I was led to believe I could never have those things. Why would anyone be surprised I ended up on the path of drugs and partying? I laugh in disbelief when I hear older straight people talk horribly about gay men: "All they do is have sex!" "They do so many drugs." "All they do is party and do drugs and have sex with tons of people." Well, what the hell were they supposed to do when straight America told them daily how horrible they were and told them they couldn't get married or have kids.

I meet young gay guys all the time, many of them 22 to 25 years old. They're mature. They're confident. Many of them came out while in high school. They're football players. Basketball athletes. They've already had a boyfriend. They talk about marriage and having kids one day. These kids aren't at circuit parties or getting wasted on drugs; quite the opposite. These kids have no clue what life was like a couple decades ago. They have only ever known a world where gay marriage is legal and they are just as capable of having a family as their straight friends. Talking to these young gay guys gives me so much hope for future generations. It is my belief that I fell into a downward spiral of addiction because society didn't give me much of a chance as a kid growing up in anti-gay America.

When I reflect back at this time in my life with the help of my therapist, I realize that the most shocking part of my story isn't that I was having so much sex at such a young age. Yes, that's alarming, problematic, and symptomatic of how society shaped me. What I failed to see my entire life until therapy was the troubling fact that older men were raping me. When my therapist used the word "rape" to describe what happened each and every time I walked down that staircase at two in the morning, high on drugs or wasted on booze, I could not agree with her.

I told my shrink, "Come on. That wasn't rape. I was fully willing to participate. I chose to go there. I chose to walk down the staircase. I chose to put myself in that situation. It wasn't rape."

We got into a verbal tussle over this. So, she gave me homework. I had to go home and find three pictures of myself as a young boy around 15, about the age I was having sex with older men in Laguna.

I didn't give the assignment much thought. I found a few pictures and brought them to my next therapy session. I pulled out the photos and handed them to her. She stared at them and then handed them back. She told me to stare at each one for one minute. She told me to really focus on me and go back to that age. She asked me, "What do you see?"

"I see me as a young kid."

She replied, "Right. A kid. Now do you think that kid you see in those pictures is old enough to consent to sex with a man in his 40s?"

I didn't need to answer. She was right. I always saw myself as a mature kid. I never once thought that 15 wasn't old enough to consent. But seeing a picture of myself and seeing how young I looked, it upset me that any 40 or 50-year-old would be attracted to that scrawny kid. For the first time in my life, I acknowledged what happened to be was in fact rape.

Rape is not about forced sex, as many believe. It is about consent. It does not have to be rough or physically brutal. It is about both people being of sound enough mind to give consent. I was not of age nor of clear enough mind to give consent.

It is not just about the legal definition of rape, although the laws are often aligned with the fact that anyone under a certain age does not have the maturity to consent to sex. The result of having sex at an early age and the impact on mental health and relationships later life is well documented. As children, we look to adults for protection and safety. What I found down that dark stairwell was anything but nurturing or loving. It was older men taking advantage of a kid. Never mind that they found a kid with a kid's body sexually arousing. It was not about gay sex; it was pedophilia. It would have been just as violating if I were a 15-year-old girl having vaginal sex.

I have no clue who the guys were. I never asked their names. I had no way to track them down to confront them. I forgive all of the men who violated me. They should have known better, but I do find myself being sympathetic to the awfulness that was bestowed upon them during their childhood and even adulthood, which created the monstrous behavior they exhibited.

2

Gay Issues

There are many labels that people can use to describe me: man, journalist, brother, addict, druggie, gay, queer… These are labels, only pieces of a larger puzzle that is Brandon. Some of these describe who I was, and some who I have always been, and some who I have become. Some are hurtful; some I am proud of. I do not regret any of them, because they are all pieces of me. Without those pieces, I would not be complete or who I am today. Let me tell you, I am very happy with who I am today, but it was not an easy road, and I am not finished yet.

I will begin with the piece that has always been part of me. I had known since I was a kid that I was gay, and that made my childhood emotionally difficult. I had no context of how I should deal with it, who I should tell, or if I would be safe coming out.

I played a lot of competitive sports, and it was common locker room talk to hear my teammates use the terms like "faggot" and "homo." They did not use these as playful terms; rather, it was one of the worst things you could call a boy. It contained resentment and meanness. It was a term to refer to someone as weak and an outcast. Every time I heard the words spoken aloud, it beat up my spirit. I was an outcast wearing a mask and pretending to be one of the guys. What if they suspected the truth? What would happen to me?

It didn't help that I was raised Catholic. Not only was I an abomination in God's eyes, I had purchased myself a one-way ticket to hell. Even though my soccer team might curb-stomp me, I would be embraced with open arms by the Devil himself.

I stuffed the shame of my existence into my "closet." For years I didn't dare open that cursed place and step out. If I had been born a couple of decades later, things might have been different, but they weren't. As traumatic and difficult as it was, the taunting has made me the strong man I am today. The only hell that exists was the one I had created around myself. No one could ever torture me more than I tortured myself during my youth.

I went to an all-boys Catholic school and later transferred to a co-ed Catholic School. It was traumatizing to hear throughout high school how I was going to hell most of my high school time. Years later, I was asked to come back and talk on career day. My response was curt and to the point.

"I will never do another favor for the school or the Catholic Church until they accept gays and gay marriage. I needed support and got none from the Church. When the Church admits they have been covering up for priests who have sexually abused children, then I would consider talking to your school."

Priests know the vulnerable children. They often tagged them with a special cross once they abused them as a message to other priests that the child was a target. It was despicable and disgusting.

Only now are state attorneys general banding together to weed out these priests and expose the Church for what they have knowingly allowed. It is too late for the thousands of boys and girls who carry that scar for the rest of their lives. There is no real justice for them, but at least they can protect future generations from abuse from these monsters.

I am lucky to live in a powerful nation where attorney generals have the power to take down the Church, but my heart weeps for those in other countries. In some third-world countries, the Catholic Church is a powerful force in their communities. They are highly respected leaders and live in countries where raping children is not the crime it is here. That is why it is crucial the United States lead the way in prosecuting priests who violate children. Later in this book, we will discuss more about the power priests hold over young victims making it more difficult for victims of sex abuse to be believed.

COMING OUT

I was living in Orange County and getting ready to move across the country to New York City to begin college at NYU. I was excited because it meant I was finally free. Leaving Orange County meant freedom, and something I could leave in my rearview mirror. It is interesting that in this current moment of my life, I feel like all I want to do is return. Return home. It is funny what time and perspective can do to your desires.

Orange County has some of the most beautiful beaches in the world. People from all over the world travel to the OC just to soak up the rich environment. But in the 90s, the OC was super conservative, so being gay wasn't okay. As I was packing up my bags to move, I had this burning desire to come out to my family. I had a fantasy of what it would be like, but I was deluding myself.

I pulled my sister Catherine aside. "I want to tell you something that I have known my whole life but have never told you. I guess I was afraid of how people would react, but now I am moving to a place I can finally be accepted. Catherine, I am gay."

Her face was blank of any shock or any emotional response, really. "Yeah, I know. I told mom you were gay when you were a kid. I have known for a long time."

That was all. No hugs. No apologies for allowing people to tease me. No empathy about how hard it was to live with that kind of secret, or how much courage it takes someone to come out. Just

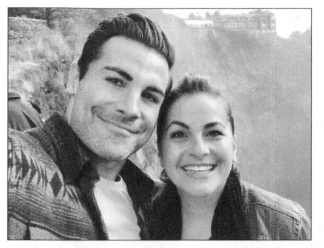

This is my sister Stephanie in

her typical selfish response. It was as if I was irritating her with the truth. She simply did not care.

Fortunately, my sister Stephanie is not narcissistic. She has been one of the most supportive people in my life and she is a champion of gay rights.

My parents were harder to come out to. I continued to be depressed throughout high school. I was living this lie, and while I had friends, I always felt I was on the outside. It wasn't safe for me to come out as gay, no matter how obvious it may have been to everyone else. Deniability became a shield I hid behind. My parents noticed the funk I was in and did what most parents do; they sent me to a doctor to "fix" me. I was sad. I was depressed. I was living a life of shame. So the doctor prescribed me Wellbutrin, and I hated taking those pills.

Pills did not erase the trauma I had already endured. They did not erase the fact that I was in the closet. They did not erase the fact that I felt like an outsider in my own life. They only dampened my senses and made me feel even worse that I was broken and that I needed pills to fix me. It was like a wet blanket on my soul.

About a week after I got my acceptance letter to attend NYU, my parents and I took a trip to NYC to scope out the campus to make sure I really wanted to move there. My mother was ecstatic because she was from Queens and was excited about me living and going to school in New York.

This trip was my first exposure to the Big Apple, and I was hooked. NYU's main campus is in the heart of Washington Square Park. It is not a campus in the traditional sense, because the buildings are dead center in the busiest city in America. NYU also happens to be in the West Village, which, in 1998, was the epicenter of the gay world.

There I was with my family, and my head was reeling as I took everything in. I was like some silly tourist staring at everything and everybody as we made our way through the city. I daydreamed about what it was going to be like, actually living there. At the same time, I was trying to decide when and where I should tell my parents that I was gay.

As we walked down Christopher Street, I was about 15 feet or so in front of my parents, drifting on a cloud, imagining the possibilities. I was people-watching because NYC is the best place in the world to people-watch.

My bubble of bliss shattered when I heard my father scream, "Don't fucking look at my son like that!"

I turned around to see what was going on. My dad was yelling at two gay men who apparently did a double take when I passed them on the street. Those poor souls had no clue my parents were trailing behind me. They looked stung. It was not as if they had said anything or touched me. I was enraged at my father.

"Why the hell would you do something like that?" I was embarrassed, but it was deeper than that. I was gay and my father, who I had not yet talked to about it, just showed his disgust toward two gay strangers. How was I going to come out to my parents now? I was mortified AND horrified. I was also stressed about the possibility that they would change their minds about allowing me to go to NYU. So I stayed "in the closet" for a while longer.

It was the right decision, because that fall I returned to New York as a freshman at NYU. I was so excited I could burst. I was free and I could be me, finally. I sought out people who gave me the lay of the land. "Where are the gay bars and clubs?"

I was pointed to the Bowery Bar in the East Village, and being a naive man of 19, I went alone. The second I stepped inside I knew I had arrived home. There were crowds of men laughing, drinking, and kissing all around me. Everyone seemed to be having a great time. I stood there like some kind of gay tourist, taking it all in. I hope I did not gawk at anyone.

I walked out to the back patio and that's when I laid eyes on him. The guy was absolutely beautiful and something stirred in me for the first time. It was passion and carnal attraction. It was lust at first sight.

He was sitting with a group of guys, and since I was a kid in a gay club for the first time, I was anything but subtle or suave. One of the other guys at the table noticed that I was alone and looking, so he called me over. He introduced me to everyone at the table, including the guy who was making my heart race a few beats too fast. His name was Billy.

We chatted and exchanged pleasantries, and more importantly, we exchanged numbers. I went home alone that night, but my head was swimming. My stomach was fluttering as I entered my dorm room. This was it. This was what my heart and soul had yearned for, for as long as I could remember. I no longer wanted or needed to live a lie. If anyone had a problem with me being gay, screw them.

Later that week I was sitting in my dorm room in lower Manhattan. I had a spectacular view of the South Street Seaport near the Brooklyn Bridge. It was a cold and dreary day, which made it a perfect day to make calls. I bundled up in my sweats and blankets. I flipped to the back of my Day Timer calendar where I kept contact information for my friends and family, and I began to dial.

I called my mother first.

"Mom, I am going to just come out and say it. I am gay."

A total, full-on heart attack would have been less painful than telling her that.

"Are you sure?" she replied. "Because let me tell you, kiddo, once you come out of the closet, there is no going back in. Do you understand that?"

Go back in the closet? Why would I ever want to do that? I had spent a good part of my life crammed in that undersized closet. It was confining, dark, and smelled strongly of hopelessness.

"Yes, Mom, I am gay."

I hung up the phone. My pulse was racing, but at least I could mark her off the long list of people I had committed to calling that day. My mother, I suppose, loved me in her own way, and there were a few times in my life that love and support shone from behind the dark clouds of my childhood, but this was not one of those times. It was her burden to bear and deal with now, because I am who I am.

She told me years later that when I was six months old and she was changing my diaper, she paused and looked down at me. She saw my smiling cherub face and my blue eyes and said, "My God, I hope he doesn't turn out gay."

"So you looked at me in disdain since I was a baby. How did you feel at four when I listened to Cyndi Lauper? And when I was five and listened to Whitney Houston and danced? Or when my sisters would paint my nails when I was nine? You just hated me? You knew I was gay and you buried it, and treated me with disgust."

She did not disagree. Only silence.

Mother of the Year!

The next call was also uncomfortable, but not near the heart-stopping level it was with my mother.

"Well, son," said my dad, "I believe that being gay is a choice, but you are my son and I will always support you, no matter what."

It was a little nicer of a reaction than the one I got from my mom, but I was still hurt and sad that in that moment they didn't show me or make me feel like their love for me was unconditional.

I continued down my list of 30 calls that day, repeating the words "I am gay." It was not any easier the more often I said it. Everyone's response was different, and some were unpredictable. I called everyone from my soccer team to every friend I had in high school. I was fortunate that everyone was so supportive and loving. Many of those I called knew I was gay, and so it was a relief to them that they could quit pretending they didn't know. I was emotionally drained by the end of that cold, grey day, but the deed was done.

KEVIN HART

They have a saying in news: "You are just 147 characters away from being fired." I'm of course referencing Twitter. We use Twitter all the time in the news business. Hell, it seems everyone nowadays has a Twitter account. Some people are Twitter trolls because they don't identify who they are. Instead they just act like ruthless and gutless jerks bullying people at every turn. Others, like President Trump, have no problem bullying people in plain sight.

Many of you, I'm sure, watched the Kevin Hart Oscar drama unfold in real time. Hart is a famous American comedian who is known for making jaw-dropping comments on Twitter. When he was tapped in 2019 to be the host of the Oscars, people cheered because it's rare that the Academy chooses a person of color to host such a big show. I thought it was cool they chose him, until homophobic tweets from 2010 began to emerge. They were horrible and not worth the space in my book, but you can look them up if you wish.

The Internet exposes everything. You think that statement you just tweeted will disappear after you delete it? HA! Think again, my friends. Everything lives forever on the Internet. Think before you tweet. Here's a good rule of thumb. After you compose a tweet, read it out loud. Then ask yourself this question: If I walked into my boss's office right now and read them this tweet, would I get fired? If you have to think about it for even one second, you probably shouldn't hit the "Tweet" button.

The Hart tweets were posted years ago, but not that long ago. To me, they are totally relevant. Hart tweeted anti-gay messages multiple times. When will comedians realize that making jokes about gay people isn't funny? Gay kids kill themselves every single day because of statements like this from Kevin Hart. Not funny. Hart should learn to be more self-deprecating rather than turn his gross humor on an entire class of people. He should know better because he's a black comedian. I'm sure he's been the victim of racism at some point in his life, and I bet he doesn't find jokes using the "N" word by white people very funny.

When these past tweets were exposed within days of his being announced as the next host of the Oscars, Hart dug in. He refused to apologize for those statements, claiming that he had addressed the issue years ago and he didn't need to apologize a second time. Give me a break. No, you should be apologizing for the rest of your life if people are offended by it. I didn't know who Kevin Hart was until recently, so I had never seen those tweets. I saw them for the first time on the news. So, yes, Kevin you owe me and my entire community an apology. Man up! Instead, Hart was a coward. The Oscars asked him to make a public apology. He refused. He rambled in an embarrassing video instead, stating why he refused to apologize. Then, after major public backlash, Hart tweeted a half-hearted apology and stated he was withdrawing from the Oscars.

While his words were pointed in the right direction, they were not enough. At the same time, I believe all of us in the gay community need to learn the power of forgiveness. People's attitudes and opinions evolve over time. And that's ok. After all, it was society who helped form Hart's negative opinion of gay people. Why should we expect him to treat our community any different? BUT, and this is a big BUT, his apology did not go far enough.

In AA, we are taught how to make a proper amends. We don't just show up and say, "Hey I'm sorry for being a real asshole. Anyway, it's in the past and I said I'm sorry, so we're all good now."

Uh, no. Not even close. When we are truly sorry for our behavior, a proper amends in this case would go something like this: "I apologize for my hurtful and hateful comments toward the gay community. I realize now how hurtful my comments were even if they were meant to be a joke. I want to take this opportunity as host of the Oscars and show the world that I have evolved in my attitudes toward gay people. I want to ask the community what I can do to make it right."

That's what Kevin should have said. That's how a smart PR crisis team should have told him to handle the situation. Hart missed the opportunity to make it right because his own ego just couldn't let him apologize a second time. His last apology was better, but again it didn't go far enough. Actions speak louder than words. In this case, actions speak louder than tweets. Spare me the words, Kevin. Instead, show me how you have changed. Go spend time with the group One-and-Ten, a group that cares for young gay kids kicked out of their homes for being gay. Do something for those gay kids who are bullied. Could you imagine if Hart—on stage at the Oscars—took a few moments and brought a group of gay or trans kids on stage to highlight their courage? Hart could have used this moment and become a real ally for our community. Instead we all just got a lesson in how NOT to handle an apology.

In the end, no one really missed Hart at the Oscars, and he became a postscript with a tainted reputation that will take a long time to fade, if ever.

WHY WAIT SO LONG?

It's the fall of 2018 and there's breaking news: Brett Kavanaugh has been confirmed to be the next U.S. Supreme Court Justice. There has been a divisive argument over the sex abuse allegations made by Dr. Christine Blasey Ford, a research psychiatrist and professor, against Judge Brett Kavanaugh that span back three decades. What did she have to gain? Nothing. What has she received? Disdain. Death threats. And the ugliest mockery from our own president of the United States, Donald Trump.

When the investigation was completed and, because there was no corroborating evidence, the FBI exonerated Judge Kavanaugh, I became physically ill. My heart ached. My stomach was in knots. I felt discouraged. I felt let down. I felt like I had relived some of the darkest and most painful days in my life.

It is imperative that you understand this: My personal opposition at the time to Judge Kavanaugh had absolutely nothing to do with politics. Nothing at all. I am a firm believer that elections have consequences and despite the fact the President Trump did not win the popular vote, he won the electoral college, and that win gives him the right to choose any justice to serve on the Supreme Court.

However, serving on the highest court in the land is not a right. It is an absolute privilege. Judge Kavanaugh does not deserve the privilege. Why? Because I believe her. I believe Dr. Christine Blasey Ford. I believe her when she says Judge Kavanaugh attempted to rape her when she was a teen. Her testimony was compelling, riveting, heartbreaking, courageous, and, most of all, truthful.

On Saturday, October 6, 2018, a message was sent to all victims of sex assault: older men in power will not believe you. Members of the Senate and even our president made it clear to rape survivors that unless we have corroborating witnesses or evidence, we are liars and the benefit of the doubt should go to the accused rapist, not the survivor.

In my opinion, they sent a message to all rapists that they have the green light to rape and assault people and suffer no consequences. Rapists groom their victims. They target people who are vulnerable and those who they feel will be too scared to talk. Rapists groom their victims so there WON'T be any corroborating evidence. Why do you think so many priests in the Catholic Church have gotten away with raping so many kids?

Because most parents would never believe even their own child if they said they were raped by a priest!

Sex abuse cases are a tricky thing to adjudicate because most of them have no evidence at all. While physical evidence or witnesses are helpful in the adjudication of cases, most have none except the word of a victim.

How can this happen, you might ask? How can people go to jail and be labeled a sex offender without physical evidence and just the word of child?

In many cases, even in the case of Judge Kavanaugh, there is usually not just one alleged victim. In fact there can be many victims, and when one alleged victim steps forward, as did Dr. Ford, others surface. They finally feel as if they might be believed, because others are coming out. There is strength and safety in numbers. In the cases of children, more than one child will often come forth as a victim, and it is not unusual for adult family members to also come forth with their stories. They can finally unburden themselves of the dirty secret that has weighed on them their whole lives.

Here are some things you should know about sex abuse predators. They are really, really great at lying. Successful sex perpetrators are the kings and queens of lying. They do it well and they do it often.

Because they are so good at covering their tracks, they are always the last person anyone would expect. Oh, no, not Father

Kent. It could not be Mr. Smith; he loves children and is a youth leader at church. How could you accuse Mr. Jones? He is a father and a scout leader! Mr. Miller is teacher of the year. Ms. Jameson is a judge. Mr. Fox is the chief of police. Sexual perpetrators often put themselves in places of power, places they can have access.

The other thing not many people know about sexual perpetrators is that they are cowards. They will lie and lie to protect themselves, but when backed into a corner, they will act in one of two ways: indignant, as Judge Kavanaugh was, or they will confess and paint themselves as the real victim, like Kavanaugh also portrayed himself.

How can a conviction even occur when you have a young child facing a person in power engaging in a game of he said, she said, in a court of law?

In my view, the tragedy that has occurred in the Kavanaugh case and so many other sex abuse cases is that because the accused are beloved and no one wants to believe they were duped—or, worse, because they just don't care--others rally around the accused perpetrator. They stand between the truth and the perception that will maintain the status quo.

What does this mean for the real victim? A scarlet letter is branded upon them as a liar, a gold digger, a manipulator. If something did happen, they were asking for it. Begging for it.

Sex abuse happens to boys, too. Do you know why they are even less reported? Take the case of Mrs. Robinson. She's the older woman pursuing someone younger than herself in the 1967 movie, *The Graduate*. If a boy is approached to have sex with an older female, they are a rockstar. They are not a victim; they are lucky. Why would a boy complain about that?

But what about a boy who was violated by another man? The shame is deep, the stigma even deeper. How do I know? Because it happened to me.

THE JADED PERPETRATOR

As I mentioned, perpetrators are cowards. They don't fear getting caught because of the punishment they might receive, although most do not believe they are doing anything wrong. They are upset because they might be exposed and therefore unable to continue their mission to sexually assault their victims. They become like a petulant child who just had their favorite toy torn away from them.

Judge Kavanaugh is a quite intelligent man. I think he has the mental acumen needed for the hugely complex job that is a Supreme Court Justice. But watching Judge Kavanaugh during the testimony made me ill. I was watching a privileged white man of power have a three-year old temper tantrum. He answered questions by repeating, "I went to Yale! I was number one in my class at Yale! I worked my butt off!" Subtext: I deserve to get what

I want. I should be able to do anything I want. It is my right, not a privilege. I earned it, and no matter what I did, or who I did it to, I deserve that seat. Give me it. Give it to me now.

In his hostile rebuke, he did something amazing. He painted himself as the victim. He took all the voices of real sex assault victims away. He twisted the confessions of victims into something dirty and vile. He made himself out to be innocent and some punchline in a plot cooked up by the opposing political party. Truth no longer matters; it is all about the spin.

As I watched and even reported these events into the teleprompter, I felt like I had been raped again. It felt like I had been assaulted all over again. I felt dirty and ashamed. The hypocrisy of statements made by Senator Lindsey Graham also made me sick. He told survivors of rape, "Well, you should've called the cops when it happened."

Perpetrators threaten their victims. Sometimes it is as direct as, "If you tell anyone I will find you and kill you." The threat can be more emotionally damaging, such as, "If you tell anyone, you will lose your family and be taken away."

Sometimes the threat is subtle and unspoken. It is an understanding that if you tell the truth, you stand to lose everything that matters in your life. These threats, both verbal and insinuated, can tie a person's insides into knots. Sometimes the only way to survive without becoming insane is to take the blame and begin to convince yourself it was not all bad. It could have been worse.

How demented is that thinking? How can one survive being violated and not finding peace after the fact? Physical wounds heal quickly, but psychological ones can take a lifetime and never heal, yet they can be even more painful than a cut or bruise. Because others cannot see the evidence, the scars of a shredded psyche, they can pass it off with "reasonable doubt."

If we can't see it, it didn't happen. If someone else did not see it, it did not happen. If you did not cry for help right away, it didn't happen. If you do cry out immediately, it did not happen. If you confide in a therapist, it did not happen. If you don't tell anyone for years, because of the threat of loss is great, it did not happen. But it did happen. It happened to me. It happened to Dr. Ford. It happens to millions of helpless victims every year all over the world.

They called Dr. Ford courageous. A hero. But what she became was a martyr in a hopeless cause, because telling the truth put her upon a pyre of wood in the town square, and in front of the world she was burned as a heretic. A liar.

Dr. Ford is a smart woman. No one gets to her position without being brilliant. She had the right kind of education and experience to know what was coming. It was not a surprise to her. She walked willingly into that platform and told the world her truth because she could not stand by and allow a man who did what he allegedly did to her rise up to a position of ultimate power which included having a say over women's rights. She was willing to burn to expose him.

I could see in her eyes that same terror and dread that I have often seen in my own while standing in front of a mirror. I know the look of a victim. Of a woman with scars so deep and painful that they never truly heal. She is my hero. Because she is me. She is a survivor, and like a phoenix she too will rise out of the flames with her soul finally unburdened, for that was the only thing she did for herself. She let the truth finally come to light. Anything else the world can say about her, to her, will never compare to the hurt, the shame, the humiliation, and gut-wrenching pain Brett Kavanaugh allegedly wrought upon her on that night over thirty years ago.

It took me thirty years before I told my therapist about the men who had assaulted me. I went to therapy because I was having a hard time understanding why I was unable to sustain a healthy relationship. I would never let people in. I had a wall built around me like Fort Knox. It was similar to the wall I had built with pillows in my bedroom to hide from the piano teacher, but this one was stronger and kept most everyone out. I only allowed a very small number of people to know the real me. But when it came to a deep, personal, emotional relationship, I couldn't let someone in all the way.

In the first therapy session I ever had as an adult, I cried nonstop for one full hour. I only uttered the words "I was molested as a child..." and I broke down crying. My therapist grabbed my hand and told me I was brave and that I would be OK now.

In the second therapy session I was able to utter a few more words: "I was molested as a child by my piano teacher and my soccer coach… and I'm afraid to tell anyone because I feel so shameful about it."

In the countless sessions that followed, my therapist asked me this question: "Brandon, why haven't you told your parents?"

"Because I am afraid my mom will grab a gun, hunt the teacher down, and kill him. She will go to prison and live behind bars and I will carry the guilt that my mom is in prison because of me. Because I wasn't tough enough to deal with the assault."

My therapist had her work cut out for her. She eventually got me to believe that I was a victim. I was not to blame. It was time for me to hand this burden to the people who were supposed to protect me: my parents.

Eventually I mustered up enough courage and strength to pick up the phone and call my mom and dad. I first called my mom and told her everything that happened. To my total shock my mom said to me, "Yeah, I know what happened. You told me as a kid."

I was furious. I had kept that secret to myself because I was worried my mom would serve vigilante justice and kill the guy, and she just told me that she already knew? What the hell?

"Mom, why didn't you do anything to protect me?" I asked her.

"When you told me, I made sure he never came back to the

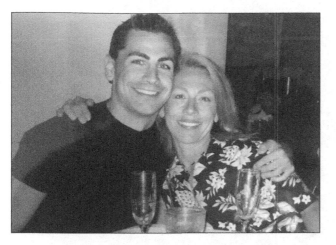

This is me
with my
mother in
2004

house," she replied matter-of-factly.

"But, wait. Mom, you didn't call police? You didn't get me into counseling? You did nothing?"

"You only told me he bit your ear..." Are you kidding me? That alone was disturbing. She did nothing but minimize my assault. That was not the worst thing she did. Because my mother never reported the piano teacher to police, in my opinion she gave him a free ticket to do it again. I love my mom and I will until the day she dies, but she is to blame for every child who was raped or assaulted by my piano teacher after my disclosure. I guarantee you I wasn't the only victim.

I get sick to my stomach knowing that he's still teaching piano and teaching kids and there is nothing I can do about it because the statute of limitations has expired.

I then told my mom that my youth soccer coach who used to

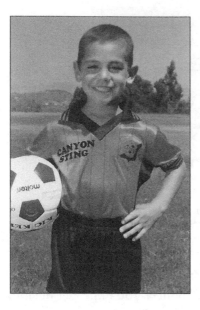

make me go skinny dipping with him in his pool. My parents were never around. They worked all the time. They trusted this coach. So for years I would go skinny dipping with him. I was seven or eight and he was in his 40s. After skinny dipping, we would have wrestling matches in his living room, naked, and he would play a game called Vampire where he would be the vampire and tackle me naked and give me hickeys all over my body.

My mom's response? "Oh, come on Brandon. He loved you. He would never intentionally harm you. Do you really think he would ever hurt you?"

Again, my protector, or the person who should have protected me, minimized my assault. I was angry and confused. Had I got it wrong?

I called my dad and told him about both the piano teacher and soccer coach. I told him every detail. My dad went into shock. He claimed it was the first time he'd ever heard about it. Excuse me? I was totally confused. I told him, "Dad, I just got off the phone with mom, and she told me that I told her what happened when I was a kid. Wait, she didn't tell you?"

My dad was furious. He claims he never knew what happened. So my mom protected a child molester and she didn't even tell my dad. That about sums up my childhood.

My dad at least told me he was so sorry that I lived through that. My dad was truly heartbroken. He was devastated.

I refuse to be silent anymore. I want every victim out there to know that they have a supporter in me and other survivors. The #MeToo movement is bringing down the white privileged men one by one: Les Moonves (CBS), Harvey Weinstein, Bill O'Reilly, Roy Moore (Alabama), Bill Cosby, Matt Lauer, the list goes on. Men in power who believe they are so powerful they can treat women like meat will eventually be held responsible. If not in this lifetime, then the time will come when they meet their creator and they have to explain why they did what they did.

Rape is not a political football. Victims of rape are not a political pawn. What unfolded in our nation's capital the week before Brett Kavanaugh was confirmed as a Supreme Court justice proved that politicians care more about power than victims. Period.

SHAME THAT LASTS A LIFETIME

It was not until 2017 that I finally came out publicly on Facebook about being a victim of child abuse. It was in response to Judge Roy Moore running for US Senate in Alabama. I just could not remain silent anymore. People were saying that because it took 40 years for someone to come forward, that in some way invalidated what happened—that, to me, was insane. It made perfect sense why those women waited years, and it was not until they had an external reason to speak up that they came out. They wanted to tell the world who this man truly was and protect others from him. The secret they and he had kept so long needed to be exposed.

For many years, I lived in fear. I lived with shame. I thought *I* did something wrong. I thought *I* was to blame. I felt so ashamed I didn't even tell the closest person in my life: my sister, my protector.

I carried that shame, that blame for decades. Even as a grown man at the age of 35, I was too embarrassed to tell anyone what happened to me. I was afraid people would look at me differently. I was afraid people would see me as a piece of used-up garbage. I was afraid people would smile to my face, but whisper behind my back, "Did you hear what happened to him? Can you believe he said that?"

It took me nearly three decades after the initial assault to finally break my silence. Does that make me a liar? Does that make my story fake? Does my story not matter because it happened decades ago?

Let me answer that for you: NO.

To those of you who say, "Why are they just now saying something? It happened 40 years ago!" Let me say these words: Shame. Guilt. Embarrassment. Vulnerability. Traumatizing.

When you doubt a victim's story because it didn't happen on a timeline that meets your expectations, you are part of the problem.

To those who finally mustered enough courage to tell their story, instead of casting doubt on them, try saying this: "I'm so sorry you suffered for so long with all that pain. No one deserves to be treated like that. I'm proud of you for being brave."

It's called being human. It's called being humane.

When I came out on Facebook, my inbox overflowed with responses. People shared their stories of being abused. They felt the darkness and shame in their lives, and they still had not come out publicly about it for fear other people's reactions.

They say there's strength in numbers. I know I feel stronger seeing all these brave men and women come forward and bare their souls for everyone to see. Some were harshly criticized and even ridiculed. My only hope is that one day, every silent victim of assault or harassment feels the same peace that I have today.

THE DOORS KICKED OPEN

In the gay world there have been rumors surrounding actor Kevin Spacey for decades. We heard about him hooking up with guys, but he has never come out publicly about his sexuality. To each his own, right? No one should ever force someone to come out of the closet if they're not ready. It is not up to the gay community to force them out of the closet for some personal agenda, no matter how much people might perceive that it is for the greater good. That might be a person's or a group's argument, but the reality is that it's nobody's business. It's wrong to put that kind of pressure on someone. Period.

My personal opinion is that Kevin's desire to stay in the closet was the result of someone feeling shame about who they really are. We are born this way, as Lady Gaga famously sings. To deny our true selves leads to destruction. I know from personal experience. I was in the closet until I was outed by a guy when I was 19. It was one of the most embarrassing and painful memories of my life.

It was a guy in my high school who had seen me at a local gay bar. I was underage. So was he. But we were both hanging out at the gay bars. He was fully out of the closet. He couldn't hide it anyway. He was flamboyant. He threw his gayness in people's faces on purpose. In my opinion, he was doing that because he was hurting inside. So when he had the opportunity to "out" a star athlete in high school, he certainly did, and he did with gusto.

Prior to me being "outed" by this kid, I was having sex with older men in Laguna Beach. After I had sex, I would often come home, stand in front of the bathroom mirror and literally beat myself black and blue. I would pound on my chest, tears streaming down my face screaming at my reflection, "You are disgusting. You are a horrible person. You will rot in hell for having sex with men! I will never ever, ever do it again, God. I promise."

Just remembering that pain as I write this passage makes me sad that I was conditioned by society to hate myself for the way I was born. I never had a choice. You actually think a gay kid WANTS to be harassed, teased, bullied, even beaten up? Give me a break. I am so sick and tired of people who claim to be God-loving Christians, yet they tell me I will burn in hell because I was born gay. Yeah, your God seems really loving.

That brings me back to Kevin Spacey. He made his first court appearance in the news in January 2019 for allegedly sexually assaulting a teenager in a bar in New England. The boy's mom happens to be a famous local news anchor in Boston. I too was an anchor in Boston and I know her and I know of her son. The boy claims that Spacey got the teen drunk/buzzed and Spacey groped him. Spacey of course denies all wrong doing. I will NOT make excuses for anyone who gropes someone without their consent. You belong locked up in prison for that behavior.

Stick with me for this next part, and if you need to sit and reflect a bit before moving on, I would suggest it. Spacey's behavior doesn't surprise me one bit. Spacey clearly has felt shame for being gay. He is one of Hollywood's biggest celebrities. I'm sure he feared he'd never land a good role back in the 80s, 90s, and 2000s if he came out as gay.

Why do you think pro athletes don't come out of the closet? Because society still shames gay people as being feminine. "Gay guys can't be athletes!" Ugh. Blame society for that. But Robbie

Rogers who played soccer for the LA Galaxy was one of America's first pro athletes to come out of the closet while actively playing their sport. I hope that more athletes come out of the closet because being gay is NORMAL! It is society that makes life hard for people who like the same sex.

Spacey had to be living in fear. That fear suppressed his true self. That created a monster, in my opinion. Mix that anger and suppression with star power and you have a real disaster on hand. Spacey was born in 1959. He is 60 years old. Having sex as a gay man during that era was an act that could land you in prison. Men during that time had to have sex in secret. That's why some gay men cruised public bathrooms and rest stops to meet other guys. It wasn't safe to be gay back then. Society forced gay men to seek out sex in these places because society told gay men that they were evil. So, when we raise people in our society to feel that there is something wrong with them, why should we expect them all to be good, law-abiding citizens? It is important to note that some LGBTQ people chose not to have sex out of fear of being punished by authorities. They chose to follow the law. You can't demonize someone for something out of their control and then expect them to live up to your standards. Again, I am not making excuses for Spacey's behavior, but I am trying to give it context. It's the reason, in my opinion, why Spacey allegedly acted on multiple occasions as a sexual predator.

3

Drug Addiction

I have always considered myself to be a chameleon. It was a survivor trait of a kid who was a victim of sexual abuse, but I also was trying to survive not being beaten up for being gay. Growing up in very conservative Orange County meant that I had to learn to blend in with my surroundings so as not to draw negative attention. It's safe to say I became really good at disguising who I was. I was not as cool as Batman or Bruce Wayne, but I did my best to keep my personas far away from one another. My gay self did not have a cowl to hide behind, so I had to create a different kind of illusion.

On the outside, it looked like I had everything. I grew up in an affluent neighborhood, played competitive soccer, and got a car when I was 16. In addition, my parents made sure I went to the best schools. My Bruce Wayne persona was easy to maintain.

But what people didn't see was the real me. The gay kid who did everything possible to deflect attention away from the real me, creating a second life to fool people and protect me. My gay persona hid in the shadows of my soul and never saw the light of day.

Being a chameleon eventually became a defect of my character. In order to protect myself inside, I learned to lie and manipulate. I did it to everyone every day, and I became really good at it. I would do anything to protect my hidden identity, and for many years I was successful. But what it created was someone who was good at lying and got away with it often. Lying became second nature, and eventually led down a path that almost killed me.

If you know anything about the story of Batman, you know that his parents were killed in front of him at a very early age. This early childhood trauma created a vigilante who worked from the shadows. He was determined to wipe crime from Gotham, no matter the cost, and rarely within the confines of the law. He had to channel that pain, and he lied, manipulated, and eventually hurt people.

When we twist an ankle, we might take some Motrin to dull the pain and reduce the swelling. But what do we take when the pain is emotional and hurts us like a throbbing tooth? Well, we use drugs, whether it is legal prescription drugs, illegal drugs like heroin, or even alcohol, also a mind-numbing drug. Each of those substances has their own level of trauma they inflict on our mind, body, and soul.

My pain was channeled inward. Drugs and alcohol and even sex became an escape for me. I had fun getting wasted with friends. Those who did not grow up in the 1980s and 1990s may not have experienced what a true "wine cooler" was. It was this soda-like drink with fruit juice and wine and was marketed under names such as Bartles and Jaymes and Sun Country Cooler, which you could buy in a 2 liter bottle. I am not suggesting that they were marketed toward children, but nevertheless, they were fruity, easy to drink, and kids loved it.

Back when I was in middle school, this alcoholic soda pop got me suspended. It was my 7th grade year and I was around 12 years old. I was the class president for my grade, which was a testament to the fact that I was an overachiever and strived to do anything that impressed my parents and family. So whatever possessed me to bring alcohol to school one day is still a mystery to me. It was, however, a foreshadowing of my addiction to alcohol and other drugs later in my life. The incident had all the red flags of someone who would eventually become an addict.

It began the night before school. I am not sure where my parents were when I began my mixology lesson in the kitchen. I found a bottle of vodka and poured a healthy amount in a bowl. I cut a few oranges into slices and soaked them in the vodka. I then placed the orange slices in a Ziploc bag and placed them in the freezer.

My parents had this small "adult" fridge in the kitchen. Inside were all of these bottles with pictures of different kinds of fruit--apples, berries, and grapes. It was fruit juice! How bad could it be? It was not as if I was illiterate and could not read the labels that told me that the alcohol content was 6%. Not bad for fruit soda, which is what these coolers tasted like.

I looked at them for a few moments. These were not for me. These were adult beverages, and I could get into trouble with them. Big trouble. So of course I had to take them. Even though I was young, I was already building a double life: one as the perfect child to please my parents and the other as a rebellious kid so the cool kids would like me.

The next morning I filled my lunch box with frozen oranges and a couple of bottles of Bartles and Jaymes' finest vintages of exotic berry and strawberry daiquiri. Lunchtime was cocktail hour for me and my closest friends. And it was my first memory of getting drunk.

I had three things working against me. First, I was drunk, so my judgement was impaired. I did not just keep it quiet amongst my inner circle of friends. I had to brag about it to everyone. Second, this was middle school, and so rumors travelled as quickly as a butterfly in a tornado. The third and final nail in my coffin was Sammy Do-gooder. I can't remember his name, but you know him. Every school had one kid whose mission was to tell on everyone in order to get a lollipop and a pat on the head. They eventually grow up to be investigative whistleblower journalists.

Sammy went to the principal. "I heard it from Tommy, who heard it from Suzy in third period science, who got a note from her best friend Amy, who said she smelled something funny at lunch, and was told by Scott that Brandon was drinking alcohol and giving it to his friends."

That was enough testimony for my principal and I was hauled into his office.

"No, it's not true," I pleaded. "I did not know that was alcohol. I saw the fruit on the bottle and thought it was fruit soda."

This, in hindsight, was another red flag. I not only drank for the first time, it was also the first time I lied about my drinking using manipulation. Unfortunately for me, I was a rookie at it in 7th grade and was given a week-long suspension.

"That's my punishment?" I asked. That was not a punishment; that was a week's vacation from school. Facing my parents was something entirely different.

There were again some factors to consider in this situation. First, I was a great student. I made good grades, my teachers loved me, and I always turned in my homework. There was a box checked off in my favor. Second, I was class president. I was an overachiever always trying to impress my parents, and they did occasionally notice. Another check. I was involved in sports and I was a top athlete in the leagues I played. Another check for me.

The final check was just dumb luck and perfect timing. The

week before the incident, my parents went out of town. These were different times in which kids were left home alone with some pizza money on the counter and a number to the hotel should the house catch fire. My sister, Catherine, thought it would be the perfect time to take out the family Suburban for a spin with some of her besties. Here's the problem. She was just 15 and did not have a license. No one was hurt or killed when she totaled the car.

I am not sure why, or what my parents must have been thinking, but she was not punished for totaling the car.

When I got home I wished for the best and prepared for the worst. I once again took the honorable road, and lied.

"I swear, I thought it was fruit juice. There is fruit on the label."

I suppose they took everything into account, like my good grades in school and they either believed me or just didn't care. After all, they had to buy a replacement car. A drunk 12-year-old was way less important than that. I sat the rest of the week at home as punishment. There were many lessons learned that day, and none of them were good.

My vices progressed fast. At age 16, I used to go stag to massive raves on Indian reservations in Indio, California. You found these raves by driving to a dot on a map you were given. There was a line of cars in the desert and there would be someone handing out another map to where the rave was being held.

I would buy ecstasy and drive for hours to party. Sometimes I would party for 48 hours straight in the middle of the desert with random strangers enjoying house music until the sun came up, only to watch it set again without any sleep. I would crawl inside the large speakers blasting music so I could feel the thump of the bass against my body.

I remember sitting in a circle of people and a crack pipe was being sent around. It was the first time I saw one, and something about the foil and the way it was smoked scared me. So I passed. I was doing every other drug known to man, but something about crack seemed hardcore.

I was in pain. I was confused and lost. The only thing that I felt could keep me sane was escape, by any means possible, no matter the personal cost. Eventually my bill came due, but it was not for many years.

THE NEW CITY OF SIN

I became very good at balancing my double life. I was able to party my ass off while maintaining great grades in school and kicking ass in sports. My parents weren't fools; they knew I was out partying, but they didn't say much because I was able to maintain my studies. I was not a "problem child" who was getting in trouble at school or with the law. They thought the worst I was doing was some underaged drinking. They did not have a clue that I had been doing hardcore drugs since I was 16.

I won't say they were responsible for my irresponsible behavior, but their motto, and one I continued to live by, "Work hard, play harder." As long as I didn't mess up my grades in school—as long as I dominated on the soccer field—then I could play hard with my friends.

When I moved to NYU, not only did I find my gay community, but I also found some serious drinking and drug buddies. Within 48 hours of landing in the Big Apple I made friends with guys who were years older than me. These were not college guys, these were men living and working in the city. I was the only guy in the group still in college.

These guys gave me access to the cool underground NYC clubs where debauchery ensued the moment you walked through the secret doors. One club we would frequent was called APT, short for apartment. It was literally a nightclub crammed into an apartment, and the line would wrap around the block. You would ring the apartment buzzer and a doorman would come outside. He would look at the group standing there and decide if they were cute enough to be allowed in. He would point at people and tell them to leave, or he would point at you and tell you to come inside. Those were the glory days of NYC clubbing, almost reminiscent of the Studio 54 days where drugs and sex were just part of the fabric that made NYC such a desirable place to work hard, play hard. Even the most successful CEOs would cross the velvet ropes for a night of debauchery.

DOSING WITH GHB

As years passed, my party friends would wax and wane. I only cared about the people who wanted to party hard. My party days intensified once I left NYC and moved to Boston, then eventually back to Los Angeles.

In Los Angeles, at age 28, was when things really got bad. I would meet up with my friends at some of West Hollywood's hottest nightclubs: The Abbey, Eleven, and FuBar. We would get to the bars around 11 pm, around the time I got off work. I would park my truck nearby and make sure I was feeling buzzed before I walked in.

My best friends had no clue what was really happening. I was addicted to the date rape drug known on the streets as G, short for gamma hydroxybutyrate (GHB). It was originally a prescription drug used to help people with narcolepsy. It has some rather nasty side effects as it can incapacitate someone taking it and induce amnesia.

The problem is that most of the street G is made in a lab. Flunkies who never passed high school chemistry used lye or drain cleaner and mixed it with GBL, which is a chemical cousin to G. GBL is an industrial solvent used to strip floors. I used to order G by the gallon from a company in the UK called Alloy Cleaner. Yes, the stuff promised to clean the grease off your rims and make them sparkle. I suppose it made my insides all clean and shiny. More likely it was corrosive and eating through my body like battery acid.

You only need a half a capful to get messed up really quickly. The best way to describe the high is that warm and fuzzy feeling you get when you're buzzed on alcohol. But too much G and you will blackout.

So before meeting up inside the bars with my friends, I would do a cap of G and wait about 10 minutes for it to hit me, and then I would walk inside the club. Looking back at my mental state, I would say that I was so uncomfortable in my own skin that I had to drink cleaning solvent to make me feel safe enough to socialize. I would order a soda water but have the bartender put it in an alcohol glass with a lime wedge so my friends would think I was drinking. It was just another easy lie and deception. Most of my friends had no clue I was always wasted on G. Those who did know that I used drugs had no clue as to the extent of my addiction.

INHALING THE DEVIL

Last call in Hollywood is 1:30 am. By 1:45, my friends and I would hug each other and say our goodbyes and go our separate ways. Most everyone else went home to bed except me. My night was just beginning. I was excited for last call because that's when

MY real fun would begin. I would say to myself, "Finally!"

I would say goodbye to my friends and get into my truck. First stop, the donut shop. I needed sugar in my bloodstream. I stopped at the same donut shop off Santa Monica Blvd in WeHo. It was tradition. I would eat two donuts, one glazed and one chocolate. Instead of milk to wash it down, I poured a cap of G into a soda. I had 10 minutes to make it to the next stop before the drugs hit me hard.

That next stop was the Flex Nightclub, which was a bathhouse. Bathhouses date back to Roman times. They were places men met and had sex with one another, multiple partners and even young boys. There were no rules or shame. It was all about pleasure without consequence, no matter how twisted that pleasure manifested.

These dens of debauchery still exist. By nature I am a germaphobe, so the fact that I not only visited them but also got naked and had sex in them is a testament to how screwed up and high I was. I always started out by doing a dose of GBH. Fifteen minutes later, all my inhibitions dissolved into a warm, comfortable feeling of bliss with an extra helping of "I don't give a crap." It was like the formula that turned meek Dr. Jekyll into the monster Mr. Hyde.

The Flex bathhouse was in LA on Melrose near the 101. It was a real pit, a dingy, disgusting, hole-in-the-wall place. It had about 100 rooms which you could rent for 8 hours at a time for

$40. You paid the guy at the front and were handed a towel.

In the room was a mattress with a dirty, used sheet on top. There was a TV in one corner and not much else. I stripped down to nothing but a towel, cracked the door, and waited. It became a revolving door of men.

If I was still high at the end of the eight hours, I would go to the desk, drop another $40, and go for another eight hours. I never remembered faces because I was too high. It was all just a blur.

I was addicted to sex, and I am not proud of what I did. It should come as no shock that I did contract a few STD's over the years, but how I never contracted HIV or hepatitis still baffles me.

On one particular night, a guy I met at Flex asked me if I wanted to go back to his room and I said yes. When we got inside, I was already wasted on G. I was feeling really good. He opened his backpack and pulled out a clear glass pipe. Then he pulled out a small blowtorch. He turned it on and began heating the glass pipe. After about 10 seconds, white smoke started coming out the tiny hole at the top. He inhaled the white smoke, held it in his lungs for about five seconds, and then blew out. Remember when I mentioned I used to party at raves at age 16 and was offered a hit off the crack pipe, but refused because I thought it was too hard core? Well, this time I gave in to the devil on my shoulder.

He turned to me and offered me a hit. For the first time, I said "screw it." I hit the pipe. I held it in for several seconds and blew out. As I blew out the smoke I looked at myself in the mirror. It was an exhilarating feeling. Within seconds I felt like Superman. I felt like a superhero. I felt invincible; I could do or be anything. I had never felt so powerful before. I think we had sex for about 12 hours straight. It was intense.

I loved that feeling so much I became obsessed. On a scale of 1-10, I felt like an 11. Over the next six months, I chased that meth high. Every weekend I was hitting the pipe.

I had lied to so many people in my life that I could not recognize that I was lying to myself. I convinced myself I was not a meth head because I technically never bought meth. I was safe as long as other guys bought it and let me hit their pipe. As long as I didn't buy the drug, I wasn't an addict.

It was an Oscar-winning performance and I was the audience. I accepted the performance and asked no questions. I am not sure if it was the drugs, my naivete, or I just wanted to find a way to feel invulnerable. That first high is like inhaling the devil. There is this promise that it will be like that again and again, and so you accept that evil into your soul. You accept the promise that is never fulfilled, and you would sell your own kidney to experience it again, and so you do more. You become obsessed. Nothing else in life matters as much as that moment the devil enters your lungs, giving you that first taste. A tease. A continued promise that is nothing but the lie we tell ourselves.

4

Sex Addiction

My sexual addiction began before I could legally drive, living at home and visiting the Boom Boom Room. My addiction knew no bounds.

One of the most shameful things I've ever done happened while I was attending NYU, I prostituted myself one time. America Online (AOL) chat rooms were popular then. We used dial-up modems to connect to the site and we could meet and chat with strangers. One of the users asked me if I had considered giving another man a massage. He offered me $300 to do it.

I didn't need the money. Not only were my parents paying for college, but I was also receiving a healthy stipend from them for any expenses. The offer was exciting, though. He did not want to meet at his place; he wanted me to do the massage at my dorm. I guess it was part of some role play for him. I had even gone to a local spa to buy some massage oil.

I met him downstairs and checked him in. He was a rather large man in his 40s. I can't imagine what the front desk people must have been thinking.

He was not an attractive man, and he was a bit creepy. I kept telling myself to focus on the money. He did ask me to have sex with him, but I just couldn't do it. I suddenly felt the shame of my actions. I needed this guy gone immediately. He paid me the $300, and I was so glad he left. I did feel a sense of empowerment in receiving the money, but not enough to ever want to try it again.

CIRCUIT PARTIES

There is an entire world that exists within the gay community that most people have never heard of, or if they have, can hardly believe it. There are few if any straight communities that can compare to gay circuit parties.

In the 1980s, when the AIDS scare began, there was little money being spent on research. There was this underlying feeling that in some way it was merely a gay disease, and that if gay people died from it, then they deserved it. There were few studies being conducted, and most of them were unfunded. Meanwhile, people were dying, and there seemed to be no cure in sight.

The gay community rose up and developed gay circuit parties

as a type of fundraiser. They would raise millions of dollars and all of the money went to HIV research. In the beginning it was about helping each other out, and the $150 tickets you bought to attend these parties were tax deductible. The parties occurred all over the world, and hundreds of thousands of people attended them.

Today circuit parties are nothing but Sodom and Gomorrah-level dens of depravity. They promote unprotected sex and heavy drug usage. Now that the HIV epidemic has settled a bit, only about 50% of the money raised is used for whatever the organizers want to use it for, and the rest is seed for the next party.

Two things that are intimately connected are drugs and sex; the use of drugs leads to all kinds of sex acts, most occurring without condoms. Men can now take the drug PrEP (Pre-Exposure Prophylaxis). It is an antiviral drug that prevents HIV-negative men from contracting the virus. I myself take it daily.

The fear of dying from having unprotected sex has become something of the past because of the mental assurance that PrEP provides. Many men want to have bareback sex with other men, which means they want to have unprotected sex. Bareback = no condoms.

The problem is that because of the heavy drug use that is promoted at gay circuit parties, men's inhibitions and judgement becomes severely impaired, and so they engage in anonymous bareback sex with multiple partners. The result is that HIV spreads, but just as alarming are the other sexually transmitted diseases such as gonorrhea, syphilis, and herpes. Again, there is little fear about these diseases, even though they have become a serious health pandemic. Many of these men get antibiotics to treat their STDs, which can lead to superbugs. These are resistant strains of diseases that are not easily treated by current antibiotics and can result in serious illness and other health complications.

Even though the official statement of the gay circuit parties is that they do not tolerate unprotected sex, that's a lie; they promote it. There is a famous circuit party that occurs every March at Roseland Ballroom in New York City, called the Black Party.

Thousands of gay men show up for this event. There are locker rooms downstairs in which men strip down to the nude or jockstraps. Upstairs are the main stage events. I have personally sat a few feet from the stage and witnessed two men fisting each other to the cheers and applause of multitudes of men in the audience and dance floor. Fisting is the act of shoving your fist into another man's rectum. I can assure you heavy drugs are involved.

Once you get tired of these fantastic acts under stage lights, you can adjourn to the maze of hallways behind the stage. This is the true "black" party because all the lights are turned off. In the ambient light men are higher than kites and have anonymous sex. There are orgies of men in the back rooms performing in leather fetish parties.

The air is thick with humidity from all of the sweaty bodies grinding on one another. A popular way people get high is by doing poppers, which is video head cleaner that's inhaled through the nose. The person gets high for about thirty seconds while suffering permanent brain damage.

This sounds like the bathhouses I described earlier, but it isn't. This is a famous nightclub in the middle of New York City during a "fundraiser" for a disease that is being spread without regret in the gay community. The gay circuit parties may be the biggest contributor of HIV in the gay population.

This just describes one party. Circuit parties occur in places like Provincetown, LA, San Francisco, Miami, Pensacola Beach, Madrid, Rio, and Berlin. Hundreds of thousands of men fly in for these weekends, get high, have sex, and go home counting the days to the next circuit party.

When I was fresh at NYU, I began going to gay bars. I met men much older than me who would tell me, "You are safe now. We're all gay. We are all friends." And I believed them.

I began hanging out with them and soon was swept into the world of those wild circuit parties. I was working at the Today show as an intern 30 hours a week and was making straight As at NYU. But I was partying hard.

One of these older men, Jeff, would pay for guys to go to the circuit parties all over the world with him. He would send a limo to my dorm to pick me up and bring me to the clubs with him. I never paid for my own drugs; he paid for it all. And I was not the only young guy. He liked being surrounded by beautiful young men.

It was dirty and gross, but I didn't care. I was selfish and self-seeking. I just wanted to party and did not care what the cost was.

I got out of the circuit scene over a decade ago, but I know some of my old friends who are in their forties and fifties have been going strong since they started thirty years ago. Still doing drugs. Still having anonymous unprotected sex.

One Sunday, in my apartment, I was coming off my high and saw a man jogging down the street with a newspaper. He stopped at a cafe and sat down to read his paper. I broke down and cried. Why couldn't that be me? That was all I wanted: to be healthy, and jogging, and reading the morning paper. I was so screwed up. Why couldn't I just have a life like that?

Like an alcoholic swearing off drinking when he sobers up, I reflected on changing my life. That was, until I had my next high and the idea of jogging to a cafe was a laughable dream.

BUG CHASING

The second time I smoked meth I was back at Flex, and the guy I was smoking with said, "By the way, I'm positive."

I was looking at the mirror as I inhaled the meth smoke. It looked as if my eyes had turned completely black. Something evil had entered me, and I liked it. I turned around and said to him, "I don't care if you are positive." And we proceeded to have unprotected sex.

I had butterflies of excitement in my belly. I liked the feeling of evil and the darkness around me, and I wanted more. I was completely transformed into the beast. No longer was I Brandon, a man with a future.

I drove two hours to Palm Springs and found a pos party. Think of it in terms of a den of vampires. There were HIV-positive men having sex with one another, and the one thing they desired more than anything was to convert a guy who was negative to positive.

A guy came up to me and asked, "Are you positive or negative?"

I replied confidently, "Negative."

"I'm positive," he responded. "Would you like me to convert you?"

"Hell yeah."

I had become what is known in the gay world as a chaser, or bug chaser. I wanted to get HIV. When I tell this story, people are aghast. "Why would you want to do that?"

First, there is the fact I was high on meth and all sorts of other drugs, so you can throw logic out the window. Becoming positive meant I would not have the guilt and anxiety of having unprotected sex. Every time I took an HIV test, it was a roll of the dice.

The parties were full of men all ready and willing to have their chance to make you a positive. I returned for weeks, then would return home and take a test only to find I was still negative.

The last party I went to in Palm Springs was the darkest and most twisted. Many of the guys at the pos parties were satanists. There was a guy in his mid-40s with a pointy red beard and muscles who approached me. He looked like Satan incarnate.

"Are you positive?" he asked.

"No, but I have been chasing for months."

"I'll give it to you," he replied.

He proceeded to have sex with me, and I was sure this would be the time I would get it. But I didn't.

As I was driving back home and coming off my high, I began to reflect on my life choices. I just had sex with a man who looked like the devil and wanted to give me HIV. My higher power, I suppose, was watching over me and had a greater purpose for my life that I was trying really hard to throw away.

One of my great regrets at the time was that I felt like I was a fraud. I was lying to everyone. No one in my circle of friends and work colleagues knew of my drug-induced life as a chaser. I felt like a fraud because those people looked up to me and put me on a high pedestal because of my accomplishments, and I returned that admiration with bold-faced lies and deceit. My cage of inner demons was full and the pain of it straining to burst was unbearable.

Toward the end of my using, I was trying to chase that first high. That first feeling of euphoria. I described it as feeling an 11 when our bodies should only ever feel as high as a 10.

One night, I was doing my same routine. Get off work. Do a dose of G. Get to the sex club and get high on meth for the next 48 hours. This time I remember sitting in the parking lot of the bathhouse. I sat there for probably 10 minutes. I watched guys walk in and out of the bathhouse. They all looked high on drugs. All of them carried backpacks filled with their crack pipes and sex toys.

For the first time in my using, I didn't have butterflies in my stomach. I wasn't excited. I wasn't happy. I was mad. I was angry. I was sad. I was the shell of the man I once was. I was empty and soulless.

A tear rolled down my cheek and I remember hitting the steering wheel in anger. "God dammit, Brandon! STOP this craziness. STOP this madness. All I want is to be married and live a simple life in monogamy! Why am I doing this?"

The next thing you know, the glass pipe was in my mouth and the blowtorch was cooking the meth. I inhaled and exhaled a huge cloud of smoke. Like a zombie, I got out of my truck, grabbed my backpack, and walked inside.

That is the powerlessness of addiction. That is the powerlessness I had over sex. I couldn't stop. I wanted to, but I didn't know how.

5

Stranger in my own body

BODY ART

The folks who watch me on the evening or morning news may not know that most of my torso and my arms are covered in ink. Each has a story and a meaning in my life. After all, I carry these works upon my flesh forever as reminders of where I have been and the struggles I have overcome. They hint at my life's purpose and the promises of tomorrow.

The interesting thing is, I am not attracted to men with tattoos. I got them because I wanted to push people away. The ink created a barrier between me and the rest of the world. It was a deflection and it was a lie. My early tattoos did not reflect who I was on the inside. They were overcompensation for the fact I was gay. I was attempting to look tough and macho.

The first tattoo I got was in 2001. I was living in NYC at the time. The terror attacks on 9/11 had just happened and the city was in chaos. I was a mess. My emotions were frayed wires and my soul was in ribbons. The horrors I had witnessed that day and those that followed had flayed me from the inside out.

I had to distract myself, and so a few friends and I joined a charity event, a scavenger hunt throughout the city with the proceeds going to help those families who lost loved ones. While this still kept me inside the trauma, at least I felt useful and that I could contribute to others who had experienced loss.

The first task on the list was that one of us had to get a tattoo. It was worth more points than anything else on the list. I was in this competition to win, as I have in most other competitive sports and events I have participated in. So of course I volunteered.

I went to a local tattoo shop in the West Village and got my birth sign, Gemini, on the back of my neck. In case you are wondering, we did win the competition.

My parents came to visit me a few months later. We were standing at a local pub in the village and all of a sudden I felt the hard smack of a hand across my face. It came out of nowhere.

It was my mother and she was pissed.

"What the hell is that? Why did you do that?" she demanded. My mother was a true enigma; she ignored the abuse and trauma I had endured, but a tattoo placed upon flesh that had endured so much was offensive to her.

My next tattoo wasn't small. In fact, it was a massive undertaking. I returned to the same studio where I had received my first tattoo, but this time I wanted full sleeves on both arms. The artist warned me it would take multiple sessions and many potentially painful hours in the chair. I told him I could handle it.

The whole project took 12 hours to complete in one session. Once I was there, I wanted it completed. Whenever he checked in to see if I was doing alright, I just told him to keep going.

The artist couldn't believe it; he had never seen someone sit in the chair that long. The truth is, I don't remember feeling the pain. It was there but I went into this trance. It was almost as if I was having an out-of-body experience. I vividly remember floating above my body while looking down at myself and the artist working on my arm.

A needle was nothing compared to the physical pains my body had endured from other men. It was a cake walk. I had been conditioned to endure pain and trauma. I survived the sexual trauma I had experienced by going into my mind and compartmentalizing what was happening to my body. It is this room deep in my psyche where I could escape. It was fortified in ways my walls of pillows could not protect me from my piano teacher. I could hide there, and all of the feelings existed on the outside. They could not pierce my mental barriers. I had learned to retreat there quickly. Drugs helped me get there even more quickly.

That internal room is where I kept all of my worst nightmares and dark experiences. I locked them away, although they found cracks and leaked into my everyday life, creating flashbacks of memories and periods of dread and terror no less real than if they were happening in that very moment. It was classic PTSD, and it took me years to realize that the real way to deal with it was not to lock them away, but to let them loose and bid them farewell. To snip the hooks they had anchored into my soul and no longer give them power in my life. It was a long journey of self-discovery, and one that I am still embarked upon.

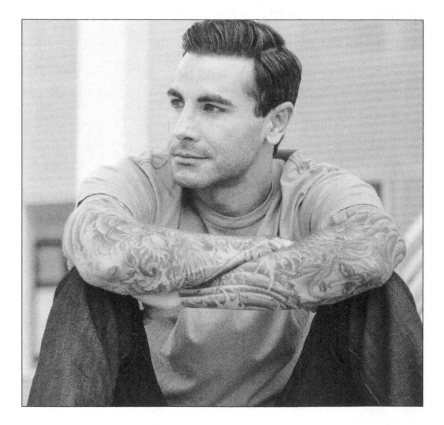

I was in a dark place, and those images leaked from their prison and made their way to the art on my arms. Upon close inspection, you will see skulls with snakes slithering from their eye sockets. The centerpiece is an image of Medusa's head decapitated. Some have suggested that this is a depiction of my mother, or perhaps the demons I kept locked inside and was hoping to someday slay. There were some dark, disturbing images, but getting tattoos was the first step of turning the demons from their internal prison and letting them out for the world to see.

Emotional pain is invisible. It is why we are shocked by the deaths of people like Robin Williams. He was a comedian, a man full of joy and laughter with what appeared to be an eternal smile on his face. Only those closest to him knew how soul-sick he really was. Even if he had discussed it publicly, people would dismiss it or even think it was all a part of his act.

People saw me every day, but never really saw me. Now I could show them my pain in a very tangible form.

Like I said, this was just my preliminary battle with the demons trapped within my mind and soul. At the time I was still a full-blown addict. That is the point people don't always understand. All the drugs and sex were like eating excrement. I had no real power over it, or at least I had lost hope and therefore my power. Hell was within my heart and burning and torturing me every day.

I was actively engaged in a war for my soul against the powerful drug and sex addiction demons. I was sometimes just moments from my head going underwater and the demons consuming me for good. I was fighting the good fight, but it was a tough ascent. I have witnessed the most determined and strong-willed addicts succumb to their demons. It is sad to witness, but just the commitment to become sober and turn your life into one worth living is a guarantee to success. It is hard to describe with mere words on paper the hold addictions have on your life. They rewire your thoughts and your emotions. From the outside it might look like a simple solution. You just stop drinking, quit doing drugs and avoid sleeping with strangers, like it is some sort of faucet you can just turn off.

Addiction claws dig deep and they refuse to let go. Even when you begin tearing them away, the claws take chunks of you with them. It's painful, and the worst screams are the ones that are not vocalized.

I was a fucking mess on the inside. A war was raging inside my heart, its battlefield existed inside my chest, and it was time to show the world what that war looked like. It was time once again to turn myself inside out.

I was fighting inner demons daily. Those demons whispered inside my mind telling me that I was worthless and useless.

I found another artist and decided to cover my entire body from the waist to my collar bone with the saga of my battle. A visual memorial of my story. I drew what I wanted and handed it to the artist. He looked at it and said, "Damn. That's badass. That's some dark shit, but I like it!"

It was a scene from Dante's *Inferno*, angels versus demons. The right side of my body is covered with angels with St. Michael, the protector, the demon slayer, going to battle to save me from the demons.

On the left side of my body sits Satan and his court of hideous, twisted demons. There were dioramas depicting scenes from my life. A demon taking a man hostage and biting into his neck. The man who is bit dies and becomes a demon himself. Each demon represented a defect in my life: drugs, sex addiction, depression, and so on.

The time it took to do my sleeves paled in comparison to the 80 hours it took to do my chest. I alternated sides; on Tuesday I was on my left side for eight hours, and then on Wednesday I was on my right while the artist inked me. Everyone's body and mind have their limits, and by the third week I ran into mine. As soon as the artist turned on the machine and I began to hear that electrical hum, my body rebelled. I began shaking violently. He told me he could not work on me and I should go home.

Remember when I said I don't like to lose? I have learned to control my body through my mind. I can even get my heart rate to drop under 40 beats per minute when I focus hard enough. I refused to leave the tattoo parlor and instead closed my eyes and controlled my breathing. I brought my convulsing body back under control. After about ten minutes, I was able to calm my mind and body enough to allow him to work on me with his needles and ink once again. I went into that internal room and held on for all I was worth, slipping into survival mode once again.

If I thought my mom's reaction was over the top about a simple tattoo on the back on my neck, now my entire torso, minus my hands and back, was covered in ink. She did not smack me, although that would have been a mercy. A slap might hurt for a second, but that pain quickly fades. No, this time, my mother wanted to jab a knife in me and twist.

"How could you do this? I gave you a perfect body. I gave you perfect skin. Why would you ruin what I gave you? You will NEVER get a job in TV! Who the hell would hire you?"

Her words cut deep and have remained ever since. She was sickened by what I had done. I was trying to show the world my pain--it was my way of expressing my pain--and she turned away, ashamed of me. My pain disgusted her, and she acted as if adding my art was a violation of my flesh and body, when the real violation had begun, under her protection, when I was a child.

Fortunately, the rest of the world has been much more accepting. I get compliments on my tattoos every single day. 99% of people have nothing but positive things to say about my ink. Many people have said that the fact I have ink makes me more relatable, more authentic. The problem is, I had these scenes injected in my skin when I was in the most pain and the most vulnerable. They were like taking communion and purifying my soul, washing away those sins. Today, I no longer need them.

If I could spread a lotion all over my body and it would erase all my tattoos, I would be the first in line at the store to buy it and use it. When I tell people this, they look at me with shock and confusion. The artwork is beautiful and it adds a layer to my image that people like. How could I want to rid myself of it?

I am no longer the scared little boy caught in a man's body. The inner room has been blasted open through recovery and some really intense therapy. I am at peace and the demons have vacated the prison I built for them. The tattoos are more of a memorial of what once was, not my reality of my existence today, or where I am headed tomorrow.

It's like the T-shirts that tout, "Been there, done that, and here is the T-shirt."

The problem is, I can't take this T-shirt off. It is permanently adhered to me. While I can see more clearly in my past for the reasons I needed to put my pain out into the world, my younger self reasons were not so sophisticated. I wanted attention as a young man, but I didn't want people to know the REAL me. I wanted them to see me as someone they wanted, not the man I truly was. I wanted to project an image of toughness and masculinity. I no longer need the costume I created for myself. I no longer have anything to prove to anyone other than myself.

The man I am today would never get a tattoo. Why? Because

I am so comfortable in my own skin. I love who I am today. What I struggle with is fighting the stereotypes that still exist with people who have tattoos. I have become a good study of people in my life, both as an investigative journalist ferreting out the truth, but also as a way to survive. I pay attention to nonverbal clues to have a sense about how people perceive me, or whether they are a threat to me.

People who don't know me often assume I'm a thug or a trouble maker. I can see it in their eyes; I can watch how they might back away or avoid me. I am not who they think I am, but because they see the ink first, I am never given an opportunity to make a good first impression.

My mother did make one prediction that turned out to be partially true. I have been passed over for jobs because of my tattoos. I will never forget when my agent at the time called me to say an executive at NBC News in New York decided to pass on me being an anchor because he'd seen a picture of me with my ink. He told my agent, "We can't have someone looking like that representing NBC News." My body art is covered every night that I am on the air, and unless I decide to share a picture of myself without a shirt, no one is ever the wiser. This man was nearly 70, and he could not handle the fact that my tattoos existed. He felt that people with tattoos are a troubled lot. That somehow the ink on my skin was the mark of Cain, or a scarlet letter of shame. The shame resides on that man, because he missed a great opportunity to have a hard-working, dedicated journalist on his staff.

Regret is a useless emotion. It solves nothing, because none of us can go back in history and change anything. We can only move forward in time, so it is a waste of time spending energy on regret. I am one of those people who believes that everything, good, bad, and indifferent happens in our lives for a reason. Every trauma, every horror I lived through led me to become the man I am today, and when I look in the mirror, I really like that guy I see staring back. Sorry, I really *love* the man looking back to me. Why would I regret all the things that happened in my life that has allowed me to fight for the guy I am now?

Have I made the road to success harder on myself? Absolutely, and I have no one to blame but myself. As an adult I made decisions including getting those tattoos, but I don't regret them. The truth is, I will never get my ink removed.

Trauma and bad things that happen to us serve as opportunities to learn. They provide contrast and context in our lives. They provide an opportunity to change. I am no longer a glutton for punishment when it comes to pain. I don't have the same pain tolerance today as I did a decade ago. The room is open, and I no longer need a place to hide and duck my head to remove me from the sensory experiences of my body. I'm so grateful for that. I'm not living life in survival mode anymore. I can feel emotion again, both good and bad, without shutting down. I'm the happiest I've ever been. I don't seek out pain anymore, and I have torn down the fortress I built to protect myself from evil.

MASCARA BOY

When I hear people say they wished they were a kid again, I have a visceral reaction in my stomach. People say that being a kid is the best. There are no responsibilities. No real worries. You get to play games all day. You get the summer off and holidays. Not a care in the world. You have a million friends, and life is so carefree.

Who are these people with the perfect childhoods? I love being an adult because I can be in control of my life. With responsibility comes freedom, and it took me many years of therapy to be able to throw off the shackles of my childhood.

My childhood memories are packed with fully awake nightmares in which I was harassed, teased, and bullied mercilessly. There were good times too. I enjoyed sports and I did have some good friends, but the shadow of my humiliation at the hands of cruel kids has created an icky spot in my memory.

When we are in the midst of traumatic events, we react, not reflect upon what is happening to us. Our brain is an amazing organ, because it acts as a parent to us. It takes away the emotional memories which contain pain and locks them in that vault inside us. If we had to face that painful memory every day, we might slip into madness or worse, end our lives in order to stop our hell-on-Earth experience. Unfortunately, this is what happens every day to those who experience severe trauma such as war or abuse. They can't keep the door closed on their vault and eventually the emotional pain becomes worse.

My mind did lock away some of the terrors of my childhood, but as I grew older, the poisons began seeping out into my life. It was not until years later in therapy that I was able to open that vault, assess what was in there, and finally dump it from my life. Once I did, that throbbing toothache that had plagued me for years finally subsided.

We all have 20/20 hindsight in which we can see clearly the events behind us, even though we could be so blind while they are occurring in the present. Some things are just too painful, too visceral for us to acknowledge, and so we pack them away in our inner cell. Sometimes this is a willful act. "I just can't deal with this right now. I will deal with it later." The problem for many of us is that "later" never really comes. It is a lie we tell ourselves, and the truth of how these buried memories can wreck our lives is often too late, and we become overwhelmed.

Sometimes we bury memories as a more automatic response, because we just don't have the life experience to provide context for what is happening to us. The abuse and bullying I endured in my youth was not something I could easily categorize or label. It was just my existence, and it was the version of normal in my life. It was not until my 30s, in therapy, that I could truly unpack all of what had occurred, and I was able to put a label on what had happened to me. Even then, it was not an instantaneous process. I was resistant and fought the notion that I was a "victim" and that "victimhood" sent my life spiraling out of control for many years, because I could not identify it, and deal with it head on.

Before I began to unpack my childhood, when people would ask me how my childhood was, my standard answer would always be, "I had an awesome childhood. I had it easy."

It simply was not true. It was just my internal script in order to deflect people from getting close. It turned off the trail that led to my internal cell. There was this danger that some day they would be able to unlock that cell and my childhood nightmares would run amok in my psyche. I would be this messy pile of psychosis sitting in some corner muttering to myself.

I was projecting what I really wished had happened rather than the reality of my life. Who doesn't want to exist in Disneyland in their heads? Where everyone is happy, and every day is blessed with a smile.

Back in the day when there were cassette tapes (yes, I know I am dating myself), I would steal my sisters' Cyndi Lauper and Whitney Houston tapes. When I was home alone, I would play the tapes and sing with abandon. Something about those tapes made me feel happy and free. I did not feel shame; that came later, as I pushed my boundaries further.

I was about eight years old when the bullying began. I was closing in on puberty, but my voice was very high-pitched. When I answered the phone people would often mistake me for my mother. Even though I would prank people sometimes, pretending to be her, it started to bother me that my voice was so high-pitched.

I would have to make the walk of shame to the bus stop and endure 20 minutes of hell before the bus would arrive. The teasing was merciless, and my two older sisters were not much of a buffer. Their older friends would call me Girly Voice or Miss Prissy. It seems silly now, but to that eight-year-old boy, it was humiliating and devastating. When I arrived at school, I would go into the bathroom crying. I would scream into the mirror, "God, please, please, please, please, give me a deeper voice."

I was also blessed—or cursed, depending on how you look at it—with dark eyelashes. I'm at peace with the man in the mirror now, but back then, I earned the despicable name Mascara Boy. Even today I receive emails inquiring whether I am wearing mascara on the air. Sometimes the inquiries are not as polite. "Why did you get mascara tattoos like Johnny Depp?" I suppose being compared to Johnny Depp is not the worst thing, but as a child, other children are not as kind with their taunts.

It got so bad that I took a pair of scissors and cut off my eyelashes. It only gave me this strange look that wasn't any more flattering, nor did it help with the bullying.

What is interesting about bullies is that, first, they are cowards.

They only target those they deem weaker than themselves. They have a sense, this way of sniffing you out, and pointing out that you are different.

There was this movie in the 70s that was remade years later called *Invasion of the Body Snatchers.* In the movie, people would fall asleep, and these pods would produce alien clones of them. The aliens were dominating the planet. The surviving humans pretended to shuffle around like one of the aliens, but the aliens could somehow sense they were not like THEM. They would point at them and make this horrible otherworldly scream to alert the other aliens that there was an intruder in their midst.

I grew up as that person who did not fit. Bullies would point at me and instead of making a screeching sound, they would say the most vile things they could to me, and about me, and point out to everyone else that I was different. This cruel exposure did some major damage to my self-esteem.

By age ten, the burden of being bullied finally took its toll on me. I was depressed and felt very small and alone in the world. Thoughts plagued me and would not release me. I wanted to die. *I can't live like this anymore. I am so weird. I am different. This world sucks. This life sucks.*

I was home alone one afternoon and I opened the medicine cabinet. I grabbed the first bottle of pills I saw and swallowed half the bottle. It turned out that it was a bottle of Advil. Since I am writing this, you know that I survived. I did become violently ill and puked in the toilet for about two hours.

Maybe God was listening after all, even through my pain and desire to end my life. My voice became deeper over time. Now my voice has become my greatest asset. In fact, I make a living off my voice, delivering the news and doing voice-over work for commercials. My eyelashes have continued to be long and lush, and I wouldn't trade them for anything. The girls at work tell me regularly that they wished their eyelashes looked like mine. Haters will hate, but I am no longer their victim.

I refuse to allow my pain to be anyone else's pleasure.

EAR PINNING

There was a time in my long career when I swore I would do anything and everything to move up the ladder in the news business. People who watch me on TV think that I have a glamorous job. They don't realize the amount of work that goes on behind the scenes. I work just like everyone else, but because I am on television, I am elevated to a standard--a fantasy as it were—that I am somehow the perfect person they see and hear for a few hours a day.

Have you ever had the experience of seeing your grade-school teacher waiting tables or shopping at the supermarket outside of school hours? It's weird, right? Do we assume they are some sort of robots that turn off at the end of the day and are pushed into some closet and plugged in for the night? They are turned on in the morning, bright-eyed and ready to go. As kids we form this strange narrative that beyond being a teacher, Mrs. Smith has a home, a family, and during the weekends and summer, might have a part time job somewhere because, let's face it, they are never paid nearly what they are worth.

It is that strange and odd mental picture that people have about celebrities at all levels, even anchor people. They think we just walk out of our houses the epitome of perfection. I know I am going to break some hearts here, but we don't always look like this. We have to work at it, and sometimes we look the way others think we should look. I mentioned my battle with imaginary mascara. That is nothing compared to the surgery I underwent because of one person's insistence that I would be nothing without it.

I really don't live the glamorous life people assume. I have been a street reporter for a good portion of my career, and that work can be brutal. As a street reporter I would live in those big live trucks for 10-12 hours a day. There were days when my film crew and I would drive 300 miles a day chasing down stories. Sometimes it would be 115 degrees outside when I worked in Phoenix or I would be caught out in a blizzard when I worked in Boston. I would feel gross, wet, cold, hot, sweaty, irritable, you name it. But when it was showtime we had to slam on some makeup, fix the hair, and make it appear like we just got out of a salon and hit the runway.

Most people in the news business dream of becoming an anchor, the person who reads the news behind the anchor desk in the studio. I have been one of those people. Even though the lights can be hot, the building we sit in to report is temperature-controlled.

I have moved all over this country trying to land anchor gigs in NYC, Maryland, Connecticut, Boston, LA, Atlanta, and Phoenix. As of this writing, I've been in the business 19 years. For the first five years, I was a reporter. Each day I would be assigned a story and would chase down leads under pressure. After all, the deadline in the news business can never be pushed back. The 5 o'clock evening news can't be delayed.

It was grueling, and I wanted off the streets and in the studio. It's not that easy, as there are limited seats and once someone is in one, they tend to hold onto it for as long as possible. Even when there is an opening at a desk, there are so many factors that go into becoming a news anchor: what do you look like? What do you sound like? How do you dress? Are you smooth at reading a teleprompter? Are you relatable? The checklist goes on. The worst part is, there is no one standard; it is all subjective. One news director may love you while the boss at the station across the street might think you're awful. When there is an opportunity to get on the good side of a news director, in order to be in line for the next opening, many people will do anything, and I mean anything, to impress them.

In 2005, I was an investigative reporter for the NBC affiliate station in Hartford, Connecticut. I was 25 years old at the time, which meant I was very young to be considered for an anchor role. I would not be deterred. I went into my boss's office and told him, "I will do anything to have a shot on the anchor desk, even if it's just filling in for a day when the anchors are on vacation."

My boss told me to audition and show him the tape. So I did. I came in on the weekend to practice and then I recorded a demo tape that next week and handed it to him. He viewed the tape and said, "You're pretty good! I will consider having you fill in at the next opportunity." I was beyond ecstatic. This was my chance!

About a month later he called me into his office and told me I was being given the chance to fill in on the 5 pm news. This was it! This was what I had been dreaming of. I sat next to an anchor legendary in Connecticut at the time, Janet Peckinpaugh. She was amazing. She was so kind to me, even though I was green. She knew I had never anchored before, but she told me she believed in me and she gave me a boost of confidence I desperately needed. I had so many butterflies in my stomach I thought I was going to puke.

I got through the newscast and it went fantastic. My boss gave me a high five and said, "We haven't had that kind of energy on the anchor desk in a long time. Well done!"

That one opportunity turned into multiple reps on the anchor desk. My foot was in the door, and finally an opening became available. They were looking to hire an anchor for the weekends. I told my boss that I wanted the job and he told me I was being considered for it. I was elated, and very positive about the situation.

About a week later, I got an email from the general manager of the station to meet him in his office. He is the person at the top of the food chain at any news organization. This was it; I was going to be the new weekend anchor. I walked into his big office and sat down across from him. We had a really good chat, and I was about to jump out of my seat in anticipation, when the hammer fell.

"You know, Brandon. I've been watching you fill in on the anchor desk the past few months. You've done a great job. You have great energy. You have a great news voice and delivery. You have a good look, *but* your ears are just a little too big and they stick out just a little too much. If you want to be an anchor, you should really consider getting surgery and having them pinned back."

I was at a loss for words. For those who know me, it is rare that I am at a loss for words. I honestly wanted to curl up in the fetal position and cry. I muttered something and got up to leave and he said as his parting shot, "You should really think about thinning your eyebrows, too. Maybe even have them lightened. They're too dark."

I was crushed. I could have handled not getting the job; that was always a possibility. And while I would I have been very disappointed, I would have arrived back at the station, head held high, and I would have moved through it. But this situation was not something I was prepared for. How could anyone be prepared? At that moment, I truly thought my career was over. I didn't have the looks to be a news anchor. I had a few choices: quit, ignore his advice, or do something about it. It was too important for me to quit. This was my life.

After a few weeks went by, I started looking online for plastic surgeons. I made a few calls and scheduled a few appointments. The first surgeon I met with turned me away. He said, "Your ears are just fine. I am not going to pin them back."

This couldn't be right. My boss told me they were a distraction. I was off to the next surgeon. That doctor told me, "Are you sure you want to do this? They don't seem like an issue to me, but I'll do it if you really want to."

I wanted to be an anchor; it was all I wanted. I already had such low self-esteem that I truly thought, if I did this, then my life would have purpose. I told the doctor to get me in immediately. And so I did it: I got my ears pinned back. Next stop, the hair salon to get my eyebrows lightened.

I showed up to the salon and told the woman what my boss had recommended. She looked at me and stared. After a long pause, she said, "Uh, sure. Come sit down over here."

I sat in the chair and she put her finger into a little jar of white cream. She started wiping it onto my eyebrows. After a few minutes I told her, "Damn, this is burning my face." She said, "Yea, it's called bleach." After about five minutes she wiped it off, and my eyebrows were burnt orange! I screamed. I paid her and left and started crying in my car in the parking lot. What had I just done? Why the hell was a listening to a 60-year-old man when it came to my eyebrows? I was a wreck.

I entered the studio, hoping with ridiculous optimism that no one would notice. People stared as I walked by. Ugh. I was so depressed and sad and embarrassed.

If you are imagining a dog getting their ears pinned back, you are not far off. They made an incision on the back of my ear, pulled out cartilage, then cut and reformed a new, smaller ear. Maybe the general manager was right or maybe he was wrong. Maybe my ears were distracting, but why do we have this standard in society? Do my ears make me any more or less capable of doing my job? I guess I will never know, but what I do know is, it was not my ears that got me future gigs; it was my ability to do my job well, and that I pushed harder than anyone else around me.

After the surgery, I was allowed to continue to fill in on the anchor desk, but I knew this was not the place for me. I had traded my dignity and self-worth for a man who had a personal opinion about what he thought I should look like. After a few weeks I made a demo reel and sent it to NBC in Boston. Three months later, I got a job offer from one of the best news stations in the country as weekend evening anchor. The station at the time was the 7th largest market in the country.

When I gave my notice to my boss and told him where I was going, he was less than supportive. In fact, he was furious. "You are not ready for that kind of job. You need years more experience."

I simply responded, "Well, you aren't making that decision. They are, and they chose me."

6

Death Comes Knocking Thrice

There have been three times in my life that I evaded death, and two of those times were of my own making. The first time I brushed death was on 9/11 in New York City.

I was 19 years old when I moved to NYU. I knew I wanted to be in media, and within a couple of weeks I miraculously landed an internship at WNBC Today, which is the local show before the national Today show. It ran from 5-7 am. I got up early every day and worked, then had most of my classes in the evening.

Not everyone knows this, but NYU is one of New York City's largest property owners. They have residences and classes all around the city. I lived in a dorm room on the famous South Street Seaport located in lower Manhattan in the financial district, less than a quarter mile from the World Trade Center. It was only a ten-minute walk.

In 2001, I had been in NYC for about a year. All my friends were gay and from the city. I was the only student among my friends. During this time, my drug use was heavy. My drugs of choice were Ecstasy, a pharmaceutical that lowers inhibitions, and Special K, which is derived from Ketamine, a horse tranquilizer. We would cook Ketamine in the oven until it became a hard white powder. We would then put the powder in bumpers, sometimes called sniffers, that we would take with us and snort the powder into our noses.

I never believed I had a drug problem because all my friends were doing the same drugs as I was; therefore, it was normal behavior. Before we hit clubs on a typical Saturday we would take two or three pills of Ecstasy. We went to clubs like the Roxy, which was hot place to go in the early 2000s. We would party from midnight until about 5 in the morning. Then we would go to someone's apartment and do more drugs. At about 7 am we would cross town to the club Twilo. It was a real shithole in the far west side. We would party into Sunday. I would go back to school and work on Monday and start the cycle all over again.

THE SCENT OF DEATH

I was fortunate to have my job at NBC. I had just started the program at NYU and decided to visit the NBC building with my resume in hand. I walked past the security guard, because no one was on high alert then. I went to the floor where they taped the Today show. I walked up to the receptionist and said, "I'm a student at NYU and I would like a job on the Today show."

She looked me over, this skinny kid from LA. "Do you have a resume?"

I handed her my very light resume which under experience was written: waiter at the Cheesecake Factory.

"I don't know…" she began.

"I will do anything to work here. I will work for free."

And so I got a 30-hour unpaid internship. My first assignment was Weekend Today with Soledad O'Brien and David Bloom.

In my second year at NYU, 9/11 occurred. It began like any other morning. I woke and made my way to the NBC studios. I would take the A or the C train from the South Street/Seaport Station. I would get off at 51st Street and walk to Rockefeller Plaza.

That morning, we had passed the Chelsea Station and were closing in on Union Square when all of a sudden, the train stopped in a dark tunnel. Everyone on the train was quiet for a few minutes, not sure what was happening.

Members in blue from the NYPD stormed our train car. I was not afraid, because let's face it, this was NY. I thought maybe they were after a purse snatcher. One of the officers yelled, "Everyone out!"

I had no idea what was going on. Everyone exited the train and followed the officers off the train to an escape route to street level. When we stepped into the bright morning, there was chaos. People were running in all directions. Some were gathered in front of a store window where there were televisions.

I could see an image of one of the towers on fire. What the hell? Someone in the crowd said that a plane had crashed into one of the towers. No one understood what was going on. My inner journalist kicked in, and I knew I needed to make it to the studio. I began running and would stop to walk to catch my breath, then run some more.

I made my way up to the 7th floor of Rockefeller Plaza. There are TV monitors everywhere and people were watching them, trying to make sense of the burning building, when the second one burst into flames. There was a collective gasp in the newsroom. What was happening? We did not live in a world of terrorists attacking the United States. The only other incident I had experienced before was the Columbine shooting. The idea of terrorists crashing planes into buildings was not registering with anyone. We needed answers—quick.

The news director stepped into the center of the room and told everyone to calm down. We had a job to do. She began handing out assignments. All cell phones were down, but I had to find a way to let my family know I was doing alright.

I went into the executive producer's office and asked to use the landline, and I called home. My mother answered.

"Mom, there is something going on here. I don't know what yet. Two planes have hit the World Trade Center."

My mother began screaming. It was one of the only times I really felt my mother was concerned for me and my well-being.

"Oh my God. It's Pearl Harbor all over again. Brandon, you have got to get out of there," she said.

"I'm fine. I'm fine. I'm at the 30 Rock building. I'm safe," I assured her.

I was so young and naive. I could not grasp that no one was safe at that moment. We had heard of Al Qaeda then, but they existed a world away. War was something that happened in foreign lands, not here in the United States. Our world has changed a lot since that day, along with everyone's perspective of terrorism and the real-world dangers it imposes. Even here, in the safety of our homes.

I was assigned to get interviews on the westside highway to be fed back to the newsroom. We were on the street when the towers collapsed. This wall of smoke began inching toward us, and we ran back to Midtown. The seriousness of the situation was beginning to sink in, and we were terrified.

After the fire died down, I decided to go to the financial district. I had my press pass and I borrowed a camera from the NYU film department. There are a number of things about that time I will remember, but one stands out. The smell. In the subways, there was this burnt smell, a cross between wood, plastic, and burned flesh. It was so thick in the air that you could taste it on your tongue. It still makes me ill just thinking about it, and its source.

When I arrived in lower Manhattan, I imagined there would be police blockades and restricted access. But it was post-apocalyptic. There were very few people in the area, and no one to restrict access. When people saw my press pass, they begged me to help them locate a missing loved one.

It was eerie and very quiet. It looked like what I imagined Pompeii might look with everything covered in ash, and time frozen in the moment of the blast. The ash was so thick that it rose to knee level. I filmed my journey through the area and came upon a Chase bank. All the windows were blasted inward. I walked in. There were papers strewn all around and overturned furniture. I imagined the blast caused panic and people hid under their desks, praying to be saved.

I worked for NBC for five days straight. Everyone did. We were short-staffed, so they decided to make me, this kid intern, a producer for the duration of the tragedy. It was trial by fire, but others helped mentor and help me. During the five days, most of us did not return home or really rest. I could not return to my apartment because it was contaminated by the asbestos released into the air. I relocated to a hotel in Midtown and lived there for some time.

When I finally did get a short break, I walked across the street to St Patrick's Cathedral. It was empty. I found comfort in the silence. I went to a pew and got on my knees to pray. The reality of what had happened became crystal clear in my mind, and emotions flooded in. I began crying for all those who had perished and their families. It was overwhelming. It took me a half an hour to pull myself together and go back to work.

I stashed those feelings and my experiences in that box I kept hidden with my other traumatic experiences. It was very crowded in there, and for 15 years I left it buried. Friends would share their experiences of that day—many people remember where they were when they heard the news—and eventually others would look to me to share.

"Yeah, I was in New York at the time." That's all I would say. I was broken inside. When I finally got into therapy, I was able to unpack my feelings. I realized I needed to, because every year after 2001, the anniversary would come around, and I would be in the newsroom talking about it on the air. Meanwhile, I was dying inside from the flashbacks I was experiencing.

My therapist helped me accept that I was experiencing PTSD, and that was ok. I did not have to act like the tough guy and pretend that it was not bothering me. I could accept the feelings as real and that I was having a real hard time dealing with them.

I visited NYC many times over the years, but always avoided Ground Zero. I just could not handle it. Then I decided to run the

NYC marathon in 2017. The day before, I returned to the sites I remembered from 2001. I was able to work through the feelings,

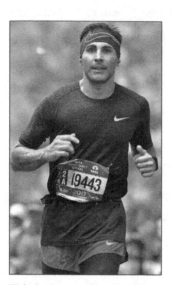

and the next day I ran through those neighborhoods and places I had avoided for so long. I cried, and in that moment, I finally began to heal.

Reflecting back on 9/11, that tragedy helped jumpstart my career. Because we were so short staffed, I took on projects that a person with my inexperience would have never been given. One of those projects was an assignment for the *Entertainers Hall Of Fame* hosted by NBC News.

This is me running the 2017 NYC Marathon

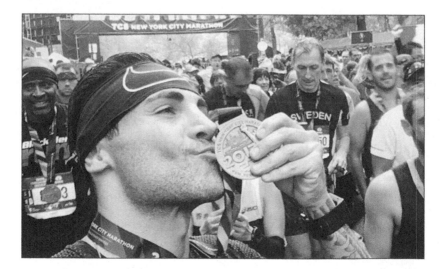

The project needed to get done, but it was an afterthought during the wreckage of a terror attack. But I was excited about the responsibility and I poured my heart and soul into it. I became one of the youngest people to be nominated for an Emmy for a piece I wrote about the induction of Billie Holiday into the hall of fame. I was only 21. Then, at 27 I became one of the youngest anchors in a top 10 market. All of this was possible because of what happened on 9/11.

It might sound ghoulish that my career took off because of such a horrible tragedy, but it's the reality of journalism. Tragic events are the opportunities for journalists to shine. Our jobs are all about reporting death, destruction, and tragedy. Yes, we do report on happy events, but if it bleeds, it leads.

DEATH KNOCKS TWICE, THEN THRICE

By January 2010, my life was spiraling out of control. In the span of three weeks I should have died a half dozen times. At least.

I got wasted on G on the gondola ride to the top of Park City Mountain Resort and raced to the bottom, only I never made it. That liquid courage sent me off a cliff, over an access road, and I landed on my head. My body went numb. I thought I was paralyzed. I couldn't move my toes. Couldn't feel my hands. I thought I was going to die in the snow.

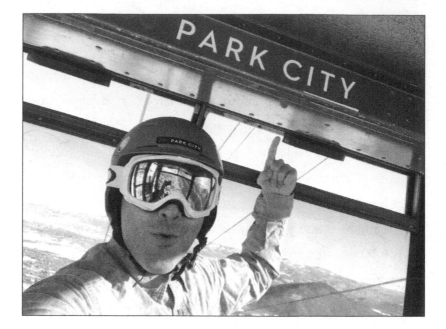

The next week I got high on G around 11 pm and woke up 5 hours later at 4 AM on the side of the 110 freeway in Los Angeles without any memory of what happened. My car was pulled off to the side of the highway in the emergency lane. My hazard lights flashed. My seat reclined all the way back.

Nothing prepared me for what happened next. I died twice in the span of 72 hours, and yet, by the grace of God, I was brought back.

DEATH'S KNOCKOUT PUNCH

One night after my 1:45 last call I went to a Hollywood bathhouse and got wasted. I got so messed up I fished out. That's the term used when someone overdoses on G and they collapse to the floor and have a seizure. It looks like a freshly caught fish on dry land gasping for every breath. I ended up cracking my head open. I was taken to the hospital and put on life support. I was unconscious for three days.

I entered the world again with a gasping breath and tried to sit up in the hospital bed. I had escaped death, narrowly. I was not alone; there was a room full of doctors and nurses around me. I am not sure if they were ready to pronounce me dead or had just completed one last heroic act.

One of the doctors looked through the ceiling into heaven and said, "Thank you, God, for saving this one."

I was alive, and very disoriented. There were bandages on my head and I had an excruciating headache. I tried to piece together what had happened without success. The chief surgeon came into my room to give me news. "Brandon, I have gone over your scans. Your brain is bleeding, and we need to relieve the pressure on your brain immediately."

I had been awake for twelve hours and did not have any visitors. To me, that was good news. Great news, in fact. I cared little for my life at that time. I was more concerned about hurting and disappointing others. That would be the worst outcome, not death. If people found out that I was using drugs, I could not bear their expressions. I had to protect the lie at all costs, even my own health and wellbeing.

"Doctor, can you understand me right now?" I asked.

"Uh, yes. I can." I had caught him off guard.

"Great. I am not waiting here another twelve hours for the chief neurosurgeon to come perform brain surgery. You can understand me, right? So, I feel fine. I need to go home now because I have to be at work tonight."

He shook his head in disbelief. "Brandon, you have bleeding on your brain. If we don't get this bleeding to stop, you could die."

I laughed a little. I was fine. I had fallen off a horse, and I just needed to dust myself off and get back on. "Doctor, you're being overly dramatic. I am leaving."

"Brandon, we have to call your family before we let you go."

There it was. Confirmation. They had not contacted my family yet. This seemed odd to me, since I had been in the hospital for three days, but it only fueled my need to get out of there before anyone found out.

"I don't have any family to call," I lied.

"Well, let's just keep you under observation for the next 24 hours and then talk again."

"Nope. I'm leaving." I sat up and looked around for my clothes.

"Ok, Brandon. But you will have to sign yourself out against medical advice. I don't think this wise, but I cannot stop you."

"Great. Let's sign it. Also, can you please have the nurse bring me my clothes?"

The nurse came in a few minutes later empty-handed.

"I'm sorry. You didn't come here with any clothes," she said sheepishly.

"Uh, what?"

"When you were brought here by ambulance, you were naked."

Clothes be damned. I was not going to be deterred or delayed; I was going to walk out that door.

"Ok, well, I will walk out of here with my hospital robe on."

It was quickly going from crazy to ridiculously insane.

"Please relax. If you can wait just a few minutes I will grab you some donated clothes."

Ever watch a clock on a hospital wall? It not only goes more slowly than real time, but sometimes it appears to be frozen or that the second hand is trying hard to go in reverse. Anxiety welled inside me as I waited. There was a caged lion pacing in my chest, looking through the bars for the quickest way out.

I knew, I just knew someone had contacted my family and they would show up at my hospital room at any moment. And then they would give me that pitiful look that would shatter my soul. I was about to run, not walk down the hallway in nothing but my hospital gown with my backside open for all the world to see. That idea did not bother me in the least, but someone discovering my house of lies terrified me.

Three hours later—I mean, fifteen minutes later—the nurse

returned with a pair of jeans, size 40 waist. (I had a 30-inch waist). She also brought me an authentic Mexican poncho. Man, I was going to leave the hospital in style. I had a pair of hospital socks to take me all the way back to the bathhouse, where I hoped my car was still parked.

I signed the necessary paperwork and took the long walk of shame down Hollywood Boulevard wearing those oversized donated clothes. I didn't care. I just needed to get back to my car. Sure enough it was parked at the bathhouse. I hopped inside and closed the door. I sat there for a few minutes dazed and confused. I didn't start the car. Instead, I opened the glove box and there it was. My escape from reality. The glass pipe with just enough meth to take a hit. I don't remember anything except what happened next. I woke up in the same hospital. The same ER, again on life support with the same team of miracle workers who saved my life not once, but twice.

Once they saw I was breathing on my own, they placed me in a regular hospital room. The door closed, and something snapped in me. It was the lock on the door that kept all the lies, the trauma, the monsters of my life safely locked away. They threatened to spill out and consume me. I was broken, and I began to weep.

I had opened my life to the evil of meth and it owned me. It was doing its best to kill me, and I was lost on how to stop it. My soul was damned and so was I.

A nurse heard me crying. She walked into my room and stood

next to my bed. She grabbed my hand and looked into my eyes.

"I know you're in pain," she said. "I know you're hurting. But God will save you. God forgives all of us. We all make mistakes, but this doesn't have to be how your story ends. Here's a booklet. You should go to this place once you're allowed to leave."

She handed me a flier to the LA LGBT Health Center. It's a place that focuses on health issues within the gay community. It's a safe place for gay people where you don't have to worry about being discriminated against. How had this woman looked deeply into my wounded spirit and known what I needed? Do you believe in angels? I just might.

The bleeding in my brain resolved on its own. Even the doctor who tried to convince me to stay for brain surgery was beside himself. He looked at the body scans and couldn't believe the bleeding just stopped. I was released later that day. Another sign from above that I was being given another chance and that I was redeemable. Although I was not quite there yet, understanding the gift I had been given—twice.

I was told to rest for five days in bed. Of course I didn't. I went to work that afternoon and when I walked into the newsroom my boss looked at me and said, "Brandon, you look pale. Are you sick?"

"Nah, I'm good. What's my story tonight?"

"OK, well, we are going to send you to the wildfires."

I thought to myself, *Shit, this is going to be a long night.*

I grabbed a pillow and hopped inside the live truck. I turned to my film crew and asked them to keep an eye on me to make sure I didn't pass out. I told them I slipped and fell and had a slight concussion. For the next three days we covered the wildfires. I remember looking at myself on a monitor and thinking, *You look like hell.*

The next weekend, I went to the gay crisis center in Hollywood. I walked in and the place was packed with other gay men. Admittedly, I was nervous. I didn't know what they were going to do with me. Were they going to send me off to the insane asylum? But, as I sat in the waiting room, I began to feel safe. I felt like this might just be the place to save my soul. After all, they were playing the movie, *The Devil Wears Prada*, in the waiting room so it couldn't be that bad of a place. Eventually, one of the workers at the health center sent me to the 4th floor, the mental health unit. I waited and was called into one of the counselor's offices. The door was wide open now. I could no longer close the door on my secret life, and it came pouring out. All of it.

"I am broken. I don't know what to do or how to stop," I concluded.

The counselor looked me in the eyes and said, "Why are you so angry?"

That was an odd question. Hadn't he been listening? I was a victim and an addict. I needed help.

"I'm not angry at all."

He repeated his question. "Why are you so angry?"

I had not started out being angry, but his repeated question was beginning to annoy me. "I'm not angry. Ask any of my friends they will tell you that I will do anything for them."

He again repeated his question, but this time didn't allow me to answer, "Why are you so angry, Brandon? People who are happy don't go on benders smoking meth, hanging out with Satan worshippers. They don't overdose multiple times in a week and end up in the same ER twice in three days."

I was exposed. The door was hanging off its hinges and he could see straight into me. It only took this guy 15 minutes to see through all my bullshit. After decades of living a double life, the facade cracked into a million pieces and shattered. I was exposed for what I really was: a junkie so out of control I should've been dead ten times over.

I eventually learned that the counselor was a recovered drug addict who at the time had 15 years sober. It was no voodoo to see how I was. I was him fifteen years ago. Fortunately, he knew exactly what I needed to do to save myself. I don't think I would have been so lucky a third time in the ER. The body and brain can only endure so much.

He wrote down an address on a piece of paper and told me, "Go to this address tonight at 7 pm."

I arrived at the address on time. I pulled up and thought, "You've gotta be kidding me. This is a fucking church."

I almost drove away, but something compelled me to park

the car and walk inside. There were two guys greeting people out front, handing out red raffle tickets. I thought to myself, *Run. Get out of here.*

I was afraid, in retrospect. This was all too real. I was about to confront a secret that I held so close to my heart for so many years in front of strangers. I turned around and started walking away.

One of the raffle ticket guys chased after me and said, "Hello. Where are you going? How are you?"

"I think I'm in the wrong place, man," I replied. "I was supposed to go to some alcoholic meeting."

He smiled and said, "Yep! You came to the right place. Take this raffle ticket and find a seat inside."

I was caught, and I could not squirm away now. I walked inside holding onto the raffle ticket and found a seat in the last row in the back corner, with my hat pulled down low to my face so no one could see my eyes. I thought I was so clever, because no one had ever tried that trick before.

The meeting began. Everyone stood holding hands and chanted the serenity prayer: "God, grant me the serenity to accept the things I cannot change, the courage to change the things I can, and the wisdom to know the difference."

A guy walked to the front of a packed room of about 100 people and began sharing his story. I don't remember exactly what he said, but I remember thinking to myself, "Dang. This guy sounds like he's telling my story."

After he spoke for about 45 minutes, another guy stood up and told everyone to take out their raffle tickets. "Ok, everyone. We have time for one person to come up and speak." He pulled a ticket from a glass bowl and read the numbers. Holy fucking shit. He read my number. The guy sitting next to me said, "Yo, man! You gotta go up there."

I was scared shitless. A momentary paralysis took over my body. I could not stand or even breathe. I mustered enough courage to break the spell and walked up to the front of the room feeling everyone staring at me. You could hear a pin drop. I stood at the podium and stared out into the crowd of people.

"My name is Brandon and I'm fucked up."

What happened next was a blur. I told them what the past week had been like for me and I ended with, "I don't know what to do. This place is my last hope. I'm going to die, and I don't want to die yet."

I sat back down in the corner of the room. The meeting ended and suddenly a mob of people cornered me. They formed a line to shake my hand and introduce themselves.

"I'm so glad you're here!" and "You're the most important person in this room tonight!"

I thought to myself, *Who are these people? And why are they so happy? I'm crying. I look like hell and these people are lining up to talk to me.*

At the end of the night I had about 50 people give me their

numbers, and they all told me to call them. One group of guys asked me, "What are your plans for tomorrow?"

"I don't have any plans," I said.

"Perfect! We will pick you up at 7 am to play softball."

That was it. That was the first day of reclaiming my life in earnest, and I have been sober since February 22, 2010.

7

12 Steps to Freedom

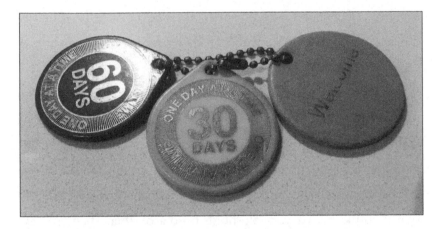

When I went to my first AA meeting, I met a group of cool young addicts. Many of them had a couple of years sober and to me, they were superhuman. How did they do it? I saw a guy get his 60-day sobriety chip at a meeting and I thought to myself, "Man, that is so cool. How did he stay sober for 60 days?"

The first step I took was walking into that AA meeting.

Looking back, that took real courage. But at the time I was so desperate to do anything to end the misery, even if that meant walking into a church to meet with other drunks and druggies.

I went to the softball game as I had promised. It was a team full of recovering drunks. It was fun. I'm athletic, so I enjoyed getting out on the field. After practice, the guys invited me to lunch and then another AA meeting. I didn't realize it then, but I understand now what those guys were doing. They were showing me how they stay sober. They were showing me that you can laugh, socialize, play sports, and be sober. They never once preached to me about my out-of-control life. They just kept inviting me to meetings, and I accepted every invitation.

It's crazy to witness how your life begins to change when you put the crack pipe down. You start to see things more clearly. The drunk fog begins to dissipate. I remember getting that first 24-hour sobriety chip. It was bright orange and it says, "To thine own self be true" with the number 24 on it. I felt so special. I held onto that chip like a two-year-old holds onto a pacifier. Then, 30 days passed. I hadn't drank once or used a drug. I got another sobriety chip. I put both chips on my keychain. I was really proud.

They tell us in AA that in early sobriety we shouldn't make any big, life-changing decisions. The reason behind that is the founders believed that any big life change could easily trigger us back to the depths of addiction. I mean, it did make sense. But 60 days into sobriety I got a call from my agent telling me that a news station in Atlanta was interested in hiring me for their morning show.

I didn't know anyone in Atlanta, but at the time I was freelancing for KTLA 5 in LA, and I had no health insurance or benefits. So I flew to Atlanta for the job interview. Two weeks later my agent called to tell me that I got the job. I was scared, nervous, and excited about the unknown. I was especially nervous about my drinking and drugging. I didn't want to lose the 60 days I had earned going to AA meetings and mess it all up. I also knew that if I relapsed, I would likely lose the job in Atlanta. After all, I had to wake up at 2 am for work anchoring the morning news. Not a good schedule for people who like to rage on booze and get high.

An old drinking buddy, Craig, posted on Facebook that he was in Atlanta all the time visiting his best girlfriend. I didn't know anyone in Atlanta, and I was moving there in a week. My old self wouldn't care because I would just plan to go to bars and clubs and meet people. But I knew I couldn't do that. So I reached out to my friend and I asked him who he visited in Atlanta because I was looking to meet people. I told him that I had gotten sober 60 days ago and I didn't want to meet a partier. I only wanted to meet good people.

Craig told me, "Wow. Do I have the perfect gift for you. I am going to introduce you to my friend Hannah. She has five years sober!"

I thought to myself "Wow... awesome!"

I packed up everything I had, including my sobriety chips, and moved to Atlanta. The moment I landed, I sent Hannah a message on Facebook. I told her I was newly sober and looking to make friends. Without skipping a beat Hannah messaged me back. "Great! Congrats! Let's meet for lunch and I will take you to an AA meeting."

Sure enough, a total stranger took me to lunch and then she took me to a meeting. The next day I got a text message from her again. She said, "Let's meet at noon and hit another meeting." I did. For nearly two weeks straight, Hannah met me at noon every day at an AA meeting. I thought to myself, "Why is this girl so caring? Why is she going out of her way to help me?'

I would later learn, years into my recovery, that Hannah was taking me to so many meetings because she was getting something out of it, too. She was helping the newcomer. I, with only 60 days sober, was helping her stay sober.

In AA you're supposed to find a sponsor immediately. A sponsor is someone with more time in recovery than you, and it's someone who will take you through the 12 Steps. I didn't get a sponsor when I first got sober in LA, and now that I was in Atlanta, I was fast approaching 90 days. That's a critical time in sobriety. It's what many of us call the "make or break" time. I've seen so many people relapse after getting 90 days. Hannah was on my case telling me I needed to find a sponsor.

She knew how important it was for me, and she knew from

experience that if I didn't get a sponsor soon, then the chances of relapse were great. Hannah is not only sober, but she also works in recovery. She helps people get into treatment. So she took it upon herself to find me a sponsor.

She told me to meet for coffee with her boss, Joel. As weird as it was, he lived next door to me. I have come to believe this was my higher power keeping me sober. I no longer believe in coincidences or even luck. Working the 12 steps I came to realize that miracles, small and big, are working in our lives every single day.

I met Joel for coffee at a Starbucks around the corner from my house. I was nervous. I didn't know what to expect. What was he going to ask me to do? I'm supposed to tell this total stranger all of my deepest and darkest secrets? Fuck that! I was an expert at building a fortress around me. There was no way I was going to let some stranger know everything about me.

We met and he asked me point blank, "Brandon, are you willing to do anything and everything to stay sober?"

Before I could answer he said, "Don't answer that yet. I want you to think about it for 48 hours and call me back with your answer."

I went home and thought about it. Was I willing to do anything he told me? Was I willing to do everything he asked of me? The answer was yes. I was helpless. I was hopeless. I had tried for so long to stop drinking. I tried so many times to stop using drugs on my own. I failed every time. I tried only drinking on weekends. That lasted about two weeks and then I would find myself back at the bars and clubs with my friends getting wasted. It was a vicious cycle of abuse. I called Joel back and said, "Let's meet for coffee."

We met up at that same Starbucks and I told him, "Joel, I am ready to do anything and everything to stay sober."

He replied, "Great! Come with me to the bathroom."

I said, "Uh, excuse me?"

He said, "Brandon, come with me to the bathroom."

I did tell him I was willing to do anything. Was this my first test? I followed him into the bathroom, and he locked the door. I was thinking, *What in the fuck is happening*? I was scared.

Joel said, "Get down on your knees."

I replied, "Oh, hell no, man. What the fuck is this?"

He said, "I asked you if you were willing to do anything and everything to stay sober." So, I got down on my knees in the Starbucks bathroom and then he got down on his knees. He grabbed onto my hands and he started saying this prayer: "God, I offer myself to Thee to build with me and to do with me as Thou wilt. Relieve me of the bondage of self, that I may better do Thy will to those I would help of Thy Power, Thy Love, and Thy Way of life." That's the 3rd Step Prayer in AA.

He stood back up, unlocked the bathroom door, and we sat back down to finish our coffee. He asked me what I struggled with the most in my active addiction. I told him I rarely drank alcohol.

I chose drugs instead. I also told him I was addicted to sex. Lots of sex.

He asked me, "When was the last time you had sober sex?" I didn't have an answer. Of the thousands of people I had sex with, I could not remember a single instance where I had sex without drinking any booze or taking drugs.

I said, "I can't think of one time. Even when I had a boyfriend, we always had a beer or glass of wine. I wasn't always wasted, but I definitely wasn't sober."

Joel mapped out two plans for me. He said we were going to tackle my drug addiction and sex addiction at the same time. Because, for me, the two went hand in hand.

"Do you watch porn?" Joel asked.

"Yes."

"How often?"

I thought about it and said, "Every day."

"What kind of porn is it?"

"Uhhh…" I had only known Joel for a short time, and this was a very personal question. I remembered my vow of doing anything to stay sober, but this was a tough one.

Joel could sense my discomfort and reluctance, so he made it a bit easier for me to answer, "OK, let me ask you this. Are they high? Are they tweakers? Are they on drugs in the porn?"

"Uh, yes. They are definitely high on drugs," I replied.

"Oh, OK. So, you watch the druggy porn every single day.

You are essentially brainwashing yourself. You are conditioning your brain to think the only way you can get off is by watching and fantasizing about two people getting wasted on meth and fucking."

That was a brilliant insight. "OK. That makes sense to me."

"Great. So here's what we're gonna do. You are not going to watch porn for the next two weeks. Can you do that?"

Easy-peasy. No sweat. I had this. "Yep. I think I can do that."

"Oh, one more thing. No sex or dating for one year."

The floor dropped out from under my feet. I had never considered this as one of the things I would have to give up when I made my promise to Joel.

"Whoa. What the heck? Are you serious?"

"You said you were willing to do everything and anything to stay sober."

It was a trap. But I trusted him. There were parts of sobriety that were very enjoyable: new friends, a clear head, control over my life. But giving up sex for a month, let alone a year, did not seem like much fun at all. I had to be honest with myself that sex had as much a hold on my life as alcohol and drugs did. The way to sobriety was abstinence. And so, I conceded.

"OK, man. I won't have sex or date."

"And… no porn for two weeks."

Taking away drugs and alcohol actually made not having sex pretty easy. I couldn't get it up. For months. I started getting scared. I was worried I'd never be able to get aroused again. I already thought I'd never laugh again or have fun again because the only fun I knew was getting wasted and hitting the bars, clubs and circuit parties. That's what I thought fun was. Fun until it wasn't. Then, fun became misery.

Two weeks went by and I didn't watch porn. I met with Joel again for our weekly meetings and he said "Great! Let's go a month with no porn."

I agreed. After a few months went by, I hadn't watched any porn, I didn't have any sex, and I turned down two offers to go on a date. Then, about four months into sobriety, I was walking down the street. I made eye contact with another guy walking past me. I turned around. He turned around. We made eye contact again. Then he started walking toward me. I got nervous. Butterflies in my stomach. I knew I wasn't supposed to have any sex, but I lost all control.

I invited him back to my place. I was sober. I had never had sober sex. He came into my house, into my bedroom. We had sex and he asked, "You smoke?" In the gay world, when someone asks you if you smoke, he ain't talking about cigarettes or weed. He's talking about smoking meth.

I said, "Nah, man. I don't." He grabbed his backpack and pulled out a pipe and blowtorch.

I was nervous and scared. And then I got angry.

"Yo, man. You can't do that here. You have to leave. Now!"

He left. I was disappointed and a little ashamed of myself. I called Joel and said "Fuck, Joel. I just fucked up, man!"

"What happened?"

"I walking down the street. Made eye contact with another guy. Invited him up to my place. We had sex and he whipped out a pipe...."

Joel interrupted me, "Brandon, did you drink?"

"No," I replied.

"Did you use drugs?"

"No, man. When he pulled out the pipe, I told him he had to go!"

I could almost hear his grin on the other side of the phone. "Then Brandon, it's OK, man. You didn't fuck up!"

I was not convinced. I made a promise and I did not keep it. "Joel, but I hooked up and I wasn't supposed to have sex for a year!"

"Brandon, I fully expected you to slip up on that. It's OK! You're working on Step Four and a lot of people relapse during Step Four, but you didn't relapse! It's OK!"

He was right. It was the first sober sex I can remember. At least I was sober, and when offered a smoke, I sent the guy packing. I had a lot of work in front of me, and many steps to go, but I something to be proud of. I needed some kind of sober sex chip or something. I had been tempted, and even though I needed to work on my sexual habits, I had conquered a big one. I had cut the cord between sex and getting high.

RESURRECTED LIFE

These are the 12 Steps of AA. I truly think everyone, not just addicts, could benefit by working these steps. It's how I turned my life around. In fact, these 12 Steps have helped me through so many challenges in my life including my own body issues.

1. WE ADMIT WE ARE POWERLESS OVER OUR EMOTIONS, THAT OUR LIVES HAVE BECOME UNMANAGEABLE.

2. WE COME TO BELIEVE THAT A POWER GREATER THAN OURSELVES CAN RESTORE US TO SANITY.

3. WE MAKE A DECISION TO TURN OUR WILL AND OUR LIVES OVER TO THE CARE OF GOD AS WE UNDERSTAND HIM.

4. WE MAKE A SEARCHING AND FEARLESS MORAL INVENTORY OF OURSELVES.

5. WE ADMIT TO GOD, TO OURSELVES, AND TO ANOTHER HUMAN BEING THE EXACT NATURE OF OUR WRONGS.

6. WE ARE ENTIRELY READY TO HAVE GOD REMOVE ALL THESE DEFECTS OF CHARACTER.

7. WE HUMBLY ASKED HIM TO REMOVE OUR SHORTCOMINGS.

8. WE MAKE A LIST OF PERSONS WE HAVE HARMED AND BECOME WILLING TO MAKE AMENDS TO THEM ALL.

9. WE MAKE DIRECT AMENDS TO SUCH PEOPLE WHEREVER POSSIBLE, EXCEPT WHEN TO DO SO WOULD INJURE THEM OR OTHERS.

10. WE CONTINUE TO TAKE PERSONAL INVENTORY AND WHEN WE ARE WRONG, WE ADMIT IT.

11. WE SEEK THROUGH PRAYER AND MEDITATION TO IMPROVE OUR CONSCIOUS CONTACT WITH GOD AS WE UNDERSTAND HIM, PRAYING ONLY FOR KNOWLEDGE OF HIS WILL FOR US AND THE POWER TO CARRY THAT OUT.

12. HAVING A SPIRITUAL AWAKENING AS THE RESULT OF THESE STEPS, WE TRY TO CARRY THIS MESSAGE AND TO PRACTICE THESE PRINCIPLES IN ALL OUR AFFAIRS.

I used these steps to crawl out of the hole I had created in my life. These steps are not static; you have to continue to work them every day, even after you have a few years of sobriety. They are the blueprint for a new life, and those who slip do so because they forget that.

I will always be an addict. I cannot drink socially or hang out in parties with drugs. Ever. They will always be a trigger, and while the first or second time I would step into that life again I might not fall, a fall will always be inevitable. It is this slope that once you begin descending, you will slide faster and faster with more momentum until you hit the bottom. My bottom was death, and I plan for that final act to be determined by old age.

Step 1 was easy. It was clear as day that my life was out of control and I couldn't manage to keep myself out of the ER. Admitting I had a problem was almost laughable because it was so obvious. Some people come to AA and are not ready to admit this. This may have been forced to go, and they are still in denial. It could be because of an ultimatum from a family member or loved one. It could even be court-ordered that they attend. They come in with a chip on their shoulder that they have not converted into one they can wear on a keychain.

Some people are not ready until they have hit their absolute bottom. They are divorced. They lose their license. They lose their job. They even lose their freedom. Everyone has a different definition of what their bottom is. One level of pain they can no longer endure.

My bottom was death. I was one of the lucky ones who was able to come back from that, with a choice. Either I got sober, or death would consume me for good. It was a much easier and quicker acceptance for me because I was not suicidal. I wanted to live. I could no longer lie to the man in the mirror. My life was unmanageable, and I needed help.

Step 2: This one wasn't as easy because I lost faith in God along the way. I grew up in the Catholic Church. I went to Catholic school. I was baptized. I received first communion. I got confirmed. I did everything except get married or wear the collar.

But over the years, I began to hate the church more and more. Mostly, because I knew I was gay, and I had nuns and priests say out loud over and over again that being gay was a sin and I will rot in hell because of it. Is it really that hard for people to understand why a gay kid might distance himself from the Church? I am who I am. I was born this way, so therefore God made me this way. How could that be a sin? Why would God do that? Did God hate me? Asking God to restore me to sanity seemed like a joke. So I kind of skipped over that step. At least in the beginning.

Step 3: Another God step. I truly stopped believing that God even existed, or if he did, he had written me off as a mistake. So I asked Joel, "How am I supposed to turn my life and my will over to a God I don't believe in?"

Joel was smart. After all, he runs one of the biggest treatment centers in America. He's been down this road with other people who argue about God. So he said, "We're gonna skip Step 3 and come back to it later. Let's move straight into Step 4."

Step 4: Whew. This was the ugliest of all the steps. This is the step where you write down the names of everyone who has harmed you. Everyone you have a grudge against.

At first I thought, "Oh, yeah. I want to do this step. This is my chance to show everyone what a victim I was!"

I wrote down my parents, my sisters, friends who had stolen from me, the piano teacher and soccer coach who molested me. I wrote down the older guys who had sex with me when I was just 15 in Laguna Beach. The list went on and on and on. I got to write what they did to me and how it affected my life.

After about four hours of pen to paper, Joel said "Great work! Now go back to page one and flip the page over. Now you get to write YOUR part in it. How did you contribute to the demise of the relationship?"

I thought, "Oh fuck. This isn't fun. This sucks!"

The lesson it taught me was this: There are two sides to every story, and even though some people treat us poorly, more often than not we played a role in the souring of that relationship.

Was I selfish? Self-seeking? Did I hurt them? Was I jealous? It was really painful work because I started to see my true self. It was so crystal clear that I had lived a double life: one on a pedestal for people to admire and think the world of, and the real me.

Someone who would lie or manipulate to get what I needed or wanted. I realized I wasn't always the victim. I played a role, too.

The only time I didn't turn the page over to write down my part was the men who sexually abused me as a child. I did nothing to deserve that pain. If I had been older, then I would have to accept that I had no business going there in the first place. However, I was kid. I was vulnerable and naive. Those pedophiles were predators—sharks. My innocence was like blood in the water to them.

Step 5: There's that God word again. Joel told me not to pay attention to the God word. Instead, he had me read, word for word, everything I had written down in my 4th Step. I did. And after I turned over the last page, he said to me "Now, don't you believe in God? Don't you believe in something greater than you? A higher power? A guardian angel?"

At first I didn't, because the addict in me always thought that I was invincible. That I was in control of everything. But after reading out loud to him my 4th Step and seeing how many times I should've been dead, but somehow was still alive, I finally began to believe that something greater than I am was keeping me alive. For the first time in my life, I truly believed I had a higher calling in this life and that's why I wasn't dead yet.

I had defied God in every way I could and even questioned his existence. (I use the male pronoun to refer to God not because

I believe He is the old bearded man living in the clouds, but it is more a matter of simplicity as a reference point.) Still, I was forgiven and given chance after chance to redeem myself. I finally did, and at the time of this writing I am still discovering my life's purpose and his plan for me.

Step 6: I was finally ready to turn all that ugliness over to my higher power. My defects of character were glaring after I finished the 4th Step. My ego. My pride. Those were my biggest character defects, and I still to this day pray every single night for my higher power to remove my ego and remove my pride so that I may better to his, not my will. For the first time I believed that my calling in this life is not *just* to be a news anchor. I love news. I have been blessed to have an incredibly successful career as a journalist. I love it as my day job. But God's will for me is to use my pain and suffering to help others find their light. Simple as that.

After all, what was the point of me suffering all that pain (some of it self-inflicted) if that pain can't help save someone's life? When I tell people that I'm writing a book about my life and drug abuse and recovery people often ask me, "Why would you ever want people to know that about you? Aren't you scared you will get fired or will never get another job?"

My answer is simple. If someone is going to shit on me for telling my story and write me off because of my past, then screw them. Judge me by the man I am today. Not my past. For I am the man I am today because of my past. And I can finally say that I love myself. I used to think that only a narcissist would say that, but I've realized that if we truly love ourselves and can say that out loud, then we are spiritually fit to help others.

Step 7: The first year of sobriety was emotional torture. It was like a crazy roller coaster ride that never seemed to end, with countless twists and turns and stomach-churning moments.

I will never forget a meeting I went to one Friday night in Atlanta. It was my regular home group meeting of Crystal Meth Anonymous. I walked into the room and it was packed. I had never seen the room with this many people. Something must have been happening that night. I soon found out that it was my friend Clint's one-year AA birthday. Many of his friends and family were there to celebrate his amazing accomplishment. Getting clean off meth for one year is a big fucking deal.

Since it was Clint's birthday, he got to choose the topic that night. He chose the 7th Step. The 7th Step states this: Humbly ask God to remove our shortcomings. The timing couldn't have been more on point. I was seven months clean at the time and I was stuck on Step 7. How could God forgive me for all the shit I had done?

We had a powerful speaker at the meeting that night. I will never forget the message she had. "If you are struggling right now, you never ever, ever have to feel this way again." That stuck with me because it gave me a choice. I can choose to work the steps and get clean and create a beautiful life. Or I can choose to be stuck on Step 7, and perhaps relapse. I definitely did not want to start all over again.

At the end of the meeting it is customary to go around the room and ask if anyone has a "burning desire." Essentially, we make time for anyone who has to get something off their chest out of fear that they might relapse if they don't tell someone. I had never raised my hand when they ask for burning desires. Even to this day, that meeting was the only time I raised my hand to share something so important. Something I had had only ever told my sponsor but never told anyone else, let alone a large group of people. It truly was like a 100-pound weight holding me down, preventing me from progressing in the program. If I couldn't relieve this pressure, I was sure to relapse out of shame.

I raised my hand and they called on me. I sat in the back of the room as always with my hat lowered so no one could see my eyes. But I have a very distinct voice, so everyone knew it was me.

"My name is Brandon. I'm an addict. I'm stuck on the 7th Step. How the fuck can God ever forgive me when for years I was giving God the middle finger? I was hanging out and having sex with people who worship Satan. How can God forgive me for that? He can't. He won't." A steady stream of tears rolled down my face.

The meeting ended and I glanced at the door figuring out

how I could escape before anyone tried to talk to me. As I was about to bolt for the door, I felt several taps on my right shoulder. I turned around and stared down at this little old lady. She had to be about 5 foot nothing. I'm 6 feet tall.

"My name is Nancy. I'm not an addict. I am here celebrating my grandson's AA birthday. I almost didn't make it on time because some guy on a bike was throwing trash all over my neighborhood. I picked up the trash and threw it into my purse because I didn't want to be late. During the meeting when you were telling the story about Satan, I opened my purse and saw the trash. This is meant for you, my sweet child."

This old lady handed me a crumpled-up piece of paper. *Yes,* I thought, *I feel like a piece of used-up garbage. Perfect. Thanks a lot, lady.* Then I opened the crumpled paper, and it read: "God has already forgiven you for what you've done. Now it's time to forgive yourself." No website. No phone number. No organized religion. Just those words.

I got chills throughout my body. After seven months of pain and tears, I finally had my "pink cloud" moment. I had my burning bush moment. God exists. God forgave me.

I went home and for the first night in a long time, I slept through the night. I woke up feeling light. I woke up feeling reborn. I shared my deepest and darkest secret with total strangers. I let it out. Doing so set me free.

They say in AA, "Don't overshare. Share the details with your sponsor." Fuck that. Don't listen to that. Share whatever you need to share to save your life. Do it to save you from taking a drink. Shame and resentment are the two most powerful things that will lead us back to our vices. Say something to someone. Don't hold it in, or it will be the thing to take you down.

Step 8: I wrote down the names of everyone I had harmed or hurt over the course of my life. My goodness, there were a lot of people on that list. People I had gossiped about. People I had cheated on. Former bosses of mine that I didn't always treat with respect. My family, even though they did some awful things, too. I broke the list into three different parts: People I would make amends to now, people I would make amends to later, and people I would never make amends to.

My sister Stephanie landed to the far right on the "never" list. I sometimes struggle with how our relationship went south. She, after all, had always been that motherly figure to me. She was a caretaker of mine. Did she fuck up and make mistakes? Yes, she did. She took a bunch of my money and invested it with some art collector and the money vanished. I held that against her. I refused to see my part in the demise of our relationship.

Eventually I took her off the "never" list. Her name migrated over to the "later" list and eventually landed on the "make amends to now" list. When making amends, you can't bring up what they did to you. This is the moment where we have already forgiven them for what they did and we are using this moment to apologize for our bad behavior. It's a really humbling thing to do. Imagine you get into a verbal spat with someone you care about. Maybe they said some mean things to you.

In this kind of apology, you don't start by saying, "I'm sorry I said this... but you did this to make me say that!" NO! We only apologize for our behavior and we ask what we can do to make it right.

Not everyone wants to hear your amends, either. I was treated pretty poorly when I worked in Boston at 7 News. My boss was not a kind person and she really targeted me to make my life miserable. In my active addiction I did everything I could to make her life miserable, too. Many years into sobriety later, I sent her an email asking if she would be willing to hear my amends to her. She never replied. I wrote a letter and never mailed it. I needed to write down my apology to her for the way I treated her. Making the amends is about me. It's about healing myself to move forward.

Step 9: Making amends face to face. Nine months into recovery, I flew back home to California to meet with my parents face to face. I took my mom out into the backyard and sat her down. I told her everything. I told her I was a meth addict and drug addict and that toward the end I had been hospitalized twice on life support. I told her how sorry I was for not calling. I was sorry for disappearing and never calling to check in. I was sorry for not being a good son.

My mom didn't cry. She was almost emotionless. I brought my dad outside and told him the same story. My dad did show emotion; he cried. "Son, I love you so much and I never knew you were struggling with this. I had no idea."

My dad was way more emotional than my mom and his tears rolling down his face made me feel like he really cared about me.

Step 10: Continue to take personal inventory and when you are wrong, promptly admit it. When I first became sober and was going through the steps for the first time, my personal inventory was long. Very long. There were so many instances in my life where I knew I was wrong, but I was too proud to admit it. Doing so would make me look weak, and that simply was not acceptable.

Here's the incredible part about this particular step: Not only is it acceptable to admit you are wrong, but by doing so you have the appearance of honesty, likability, affability, and being humble. We often become embarrassed when we believe something so strongly, only to later learn that we had it all wrong. To admit that is a strength, not a weakness.

When you admit you were wrong, it gives other people an opportunity to continue working and communicating with you. If you are someone who refuses to admit defeat or wrongdoing, no one will want to work with you because… what's the point?

A clear example of this occurred when I walked into the

newsroom one day and one of my producers made a mistake. I read that mistake on TV in front of tens of thousands of viewers. I was accountable to those viewers, and I took that very seriously. During commercial I ripped into my producer because the mistake was careless. When I'm on the anchor desk, even during commercial break, everyone in the control room can hear me. The floor crew can hear me. My co-anchor could certainly hear me putting the producer through the shredder.

The truth is while they were important issues that needed addressing, my delivery was abusive. Immediately after I finished speaking my truth to my producer, I felt terrible. I knew in my gut I had let my emotions get the best of me. I was mad at myself for not using all the tools I had learned in AA to handle stressful situations with class.

The 10th Step allows me to make amends immediately. After the show ended, I pulled my producer aside and said, "I want to apologize for calling you out knowing everyone could hear what I was saying. I should have waited to talk with you in private. For that, I apologize."

My producer said, "Brandon, don't worry about it. I'm sorry for being so careless. I should have done a better job fact-checking before I approved the script." How beautiful is that. When I admit my fault, it makes the other person less defensive and it sets the stage for them to take accountability for their actions without my calling them out again in the apology.

Even with my best intentions I could have blown it by saying, "I shouldn't have called you out publicly, but you need to do a better job getting your facts right. It's my face on TV and viewers at home blame me, not you!"

When we make an amends, we only address our side of the street. We do not call the other person out during an apology for our behavior. They may have made a crucial mistake, but we are responsible for our own actions.

I've lost my cool with bank operators, medical offices, you name it. I've been frustrated and acted out in anger in my past. It's crazy to see the change in me. I handle these situations so differently now. First and foremost, I never call a bank, doctor's office, or anything else unpleasant unless I am in a calm state of mind. If I'm hangry, forget about it. If I'm on edge or anxious, I save the call for another day, or I say a prayer and try to calm myself.

I remember one instance when a doctor's office was trying to bill me for something that never happened. I knew I was right, but they didn't care. They were threatening collections on me. I was really proud how I handled it.

"I did not have this procedure done. It is not my responsibility for this. I am starting to get frustrated, so I am going to hang up and call back tomorrow to work this out."

I don't like to admit my faults. Who does? I don't like to have to say, "I apologize." So, instead of getting to that point, I bail. I do everything I can to NOT make an amends. That means I'm taking action instead of reacting.

Dear Linda,

I hope this message finds you well, and I hope that you are open to receiving it.

I want to apologize for my behavior when I worked for you in Boston. I was defiant and manipulative into getting my way, which I believed was the right and only way. I was very selfish and self-seeking in the way I acted toward you on many occasions. I didn't think of the 7 News team first. I thought of myself first, and didn't much care of the consequences after. I apologize for not being more open to your critiques of my work. Instead, I was self-righteous. I was wrong for how I handled myself on many occasions, unable and simply unwilling to communicate with you as any good employee would. You gave me an opportunity of a lifetime, and I simply took it for granted without any sense of gratitude. As matter of fact, I simply was not a "good soldier" in the newsroom.

I have struggled with this for many years.

I remember the last thing you said to me in your office: That you believed I had so much talent, and so much potential, but I was not a good fit for the newsroom. Truth is, with my attitude at the time, I was not a good fit for any newsroom.

I have grown a lot since then. I wish I could go back in time and be the man I am today, working for you. I wish I could go back in time and be the leader in the newsroom for you, as I am today.

I learned so much about the business while working for you and 7 News. So much of who I am today as an anchor and journalist is credit to what I learned from you in the newsroom. For that, I am so grateful.

I am grateful and blessed to have had the opportunity to work at 7 News.

Please, let me know if there is anything I can do, to right these wrongs.

Sincerely,

Brandon Lee

Step 11: When we engage in prayer and meditation to improve our conscious contact with God, we can begin to understand Him. We pray only to increase our knowledge of His will for us and the power to carry that out.

This step brings me back to when I started AA. My first sponsor asked me, "How is your relationship with God?"

He then asked me to begin praying every night and every

morning. I had to pray to a God I didn't believe in. Eventually, through working the steps a total of five times, I finally got it. The 11th Step says, "praying only for knowledge of His will for us…"

Read that again: His will for us." It is not about our will. It is about His will. I have spent so many nights praying for stuff that I wanted.

"God, please let me get the job at CBS News. I really want it."

"God, please get me a job out of Phoenix."

"God, please let me sell this painting so I can pay for my vacation."

None of that is God's will. After understanding the true essence of this step my prayers are more like, "God, thank you for keeping me healthy. Thank you for all the blessings in my life: art, the beach, friends, a car, a roof over my head."

"God, please allow me to be open to my next journey, wherever that path may lead."

"God, I'm not sure what direction to take my life, but I only ask that you make the decision obvious for me."

In these latter examples, I am praying for specific things. I am praying that God put me where I need to be. That's turning my life and will over to my higher power. Remember, my higher power kept me alive multiple times when my own instincts would have killed me. Why should I trust myself, when my own instincts almost got me killed ten times over? Why not turn to the person/thing/ spirituality that saved me? I was kept alive for a greater purpose.

You really think my life "purpose" is to read a teleprompter on the news? Hardly! That is a means to end. It is just one of the things I do; it does not define who I am.

I love my career. I love sharing people's stories. I love making a difference in my local community. God's will for me is to be an example that no matter how far down the scale I have gone, I can still survive and turn my life around. God's will for me is to inspire people to achieve their best, even if the cards have been stacked against them. God's will for me is to share openly my story about addiction and being a victim of child sex abuse, so that others won't feel the need to suffer in silence. The extra blessing is that God did give me the unique talent to be a good news journalist, and I am so grateful for my career. Even so, it is not his will for me.

When we pray in this manner it allows us to share our pain with someone or something. When we speak it out loud, it takes some of the power away from it. How cool is it that I get to turn my problems over to God? Sometimes things are out of my control, but being the control freak I am, I do everything to try to control the situation in my favor. Trying to control situations and even people in this way can send us into a tailspin and eventually a fiery crash.

When we realize something is out of our control—maybe it's a job, or maybe it's a relationship when the other person shares that they're not in love with you anymore—those are the times when I pray, "God, I'm not sure how to handle this. I love him, but he says he is not in love with me. Just give me the strength to walk through this and respect him while also respecting me. God, comfort me."

Before I embraced the 11th step I may have said, "God, please make him like me. I don't know what I will do if we are not together!"

How selfish is that? That's not taking into consideration someone else's point of view or feelings. That's only caring about me. Not about them and their relationship with God.

Step 12: Having had a spiritual awakening as the result of these steps, in this final step we try to carry this message and to practice these principles in all our affairs. This is the most important step for any addict. In order to keep sobriety, we have to give it. We have to give back by helping others in recovery.

I have had close to 40 sponsees since I got sober back in 2010. They have been mostly people who are newly sober. I don't work with them for their sole benefit. I work for them for me. It's about keeping me sober.

There have been times where I've had drama in my life and I was scheduled to work with a sponsee that same day. My instinct says, *Fuck it. Cancel the meeting. I don't want to work with him today.* But the truth from years of experience is that when I show up and keep my commitments to help another addict, my problems go away, at least for that hour. It affords me an opportunity to get out of my head. It allows my wheels to stop spinning. For an addict, spinning wheels can lead to a relapse.

Every single time I have wanted to cancel a meeting with a sponsee but still met with them, I have always walked away feeling relieved. My anxiety melts away. I have a new perspective. "Fuck, I thought I had a bad day. Shit, he's really having some problems." Nothing better than a little perspective from someone who has it rougher than you.

THE CRACKED MIRROR

In my youth I was athletic. From the time I could walk, my parents had me playing soccer. I was good at it and played on club teams and was able to travel to Paris, Sweden, Italy, and just about the entire continental United States. By the time I reached high school I was not only playing on a soccer team that won state titles, but I also started to run cross country. I had the perfect frame for it; I was lean and I was fast. No matter what I tried, I could not gain weight or bulk my muscles.

Fast forward to New York City. I was like a kid in a candy shop. I finally found a place to be free. To be me. I came out of the closet to everyone I knew at the time. It only took about two weeks in the city before I began saying to myself, "I have found my people!"

There were some hot gay clubs in Manhattan. At one on the west side called The Roxy, the line to get inside wrapped around the block. I was in awe of the men standing in line. They were gorgeous. They could have been Greek Gods chiseled out of granite. Even though I was underage, I knew the doorman and was let in. If you were a decent-looking guy going into a gay club, you never were hassled or made to show an ID. The fact I was a young gay man on the prowl was all the ID I needed.

I have vague recollections of my time in the gay clubs in New York, because I was high on ecstasy most of the time. One night, as we were ordering drinks at a nightclub, one of my friends said to me, "Open your mouth, quick!"

I obediently, I mean stupidly, did as he asked. He popped something on my tongue, and I swallowed.

Then I asked him what he had given me.

"Ecstasy! You're gonna love it. Give it about 20 minutes."

As I waited for the drugs to kick in, I looked to my right and froze. I saw a sea of half-naked men, standing together like gladiators ready for their turn in the arena. Their massive muscles bulged under their skin and what little clothes they were wearing. They could move boulders; I could move fast. I was still this thin, scrawny kid, and I may as well have been invisible as none of them seemed to notice me.

Years passed, and after hundreds of circuit parties in which I continued to be looked over, I finally said "screw it." It was not as though I was out of shape, I just did not look like them. I wanted to look like them. I needed to look like them. I wanted to be one of them. I wanted to be desired by them. And, so I did what many of them did: I went online and ordered illegal steroids.

I had no clue what I was buying or who I was buying it from. I didn't care. I just wanted attention from other gay guys and I truly felt like I would never get that attention as a skinny kid. I needed to be big. Unnaturally big. I was going to be that big even if it killed me.

Imagine my delight when an unmarked, padded envelope arrived a week later. Inside was what I assumed were steroids in hermetically sealed glass vials with rubber ports on top to insert a needle. This was like getting Chinese takeout; everything I would need was in the envelope. Instead of chopsticks and a fortune cookie, there were needles and syringes.

I wasn't afraid of needles or pain at the point in my life. But I had no idea how to inject the needle into my skin, so I did what anyone else would do in a similar situation: I Googled it. I suggest that no one reading this should ever attempt to do any medical procedure on themselves by Googling it. I stuck the needle into my upper butt cheek. I bled so much I freaked out. I obviously had done it wrong. But with many more years of practice, I became a pro. Not one of my proudest accomplishments, I can assure you. What I didn't realize is that choosing to inject myself with steroids was just the beginning of a new war within myself: body shame.

BODY DYSMORPHIA

Two people can look at the same object and report what they see, and it will sound like they are talking about something totally different. The sensory input is the same: light bouncing from the image passes through the lens of the eye, hits the retina, and information is sent to the brain via the optic nerve. This is the same for most living creatures.

What is unique is the way we interpret that image. Not only what we are seeing, but how we feel about what we are seeing. Our emotions and how we interpret the world around us can change how we interpret what we are witnessing.

This is a simplistic explanation of body dysmorphia. The way I interpreted the body I saw in the mirror was tainted by my emotions concerning my body. It was like looking at my body in a funhouse mirror, all out of proportion and not anchored in reality. The image I saw was too small. Too weak. Not desirable enough. The steroids were just the beginning of my twisted hate affair with my body. It was unhealthy. It was dysfunctional. And I was never satisfied. I wanted to love the image looking back at me, but I had to constantly try to change it and improve it.

The steroids did allow me to start gaining weight. In addition, I began drinking protein shakes that had about 3000 calories in them. I was like this deflated balloon, and I was filling it with water. My stomach was a mess as I jammed more and more calories into my small frame. Sure, I got bigger, and most of the weight I was gaining was water weight, but I didn't care.

I started at 155 pounds and eventually the scale tipped at 205 pounds. The steroids and the super shakes helped me in my quest to be noticed, because the bigger guys did start to pay attention to me.

Unfortunately, I had essentially put on a Halloween latex body suit. I was still the skinny boy trapped inside this enormous body, and it felt fake. It felt wrong. I was miserable in my own skin. I had created a new reality that I began hating more than the old one.

2010 marks the year I got sober from drugs and alcohol. I continued to use steroids every day, because in my mind it was not the same as the other illegal drugs I had been taking. I had to clear my mind enough and be sober enough to be able to peel back one issue at a time. I could not take on all of things in my life that needed to change all at once. Everything has a season, and a time. Battling my body dysmorphia was my new challenge in recovery in 2012.

At the time I had an incredible sponsor named CeCe. She knew the excuses. She knew the arguments, and she was not going to let me get away with anything. She was an ex-body builder and ex-military, a true badass.

"What do you want to focus on this year in recovery" she asked.

I no longer craved drugs and alcohol the way I once did. Because I had done some internal work, I realized that I had some serious body image issues. It was time to deal with them.

"I want to be able to look in the mirror and love the image staring back at me," I answered simply. I came clean with CeCe about my steroid use and 3000-calorie shakes. I admitted that I was buying steroids online from unknown sources, so I could not be sure what exactly I was injecting into my body. I wanted to stop the madness in my life.

"Brandon, how long have you been using steroids?"

"About 10 years."

"Okay, in those 10 years, was there ever a time when you looked in the mirror and said 'wow, I finally look the way I've wanted to look?'" she asked. It was a rhetorical question because she already knew the answer. She was merely giving me the opportunity to be honest with myself.

I sat with the question. It was a straightforward question, but the answer was complicated. The complication was that I did not know what the answer was, or that there could be more than one possible answer. The complication was all of the emotions that had built up behind it. The shame. The depression. The needing to be wanted. Over the 10 years I knew I would not be happy with the suit I was wearing, but continued because it was easier than taking the chance that I would love the true body that lie beneath the facade. I had hated my body for the wrong reasons, and what I have come to understand is that there is never a reason to hate your body. I had to learn to love the person inside that body, because it was the Brandon beneath all of it that had struggled for so long.

My body had been sexually abused. Because the abuse had occurred when I was so young, I began to equate it with love. For someone to use my body meant that I was accepted. Even if they abused my body, they must care for me. Because no one stopped them from abusing me, it must have been right for them to do so.

In my sordid hate affair with my body, I had been abusing it and had convinced myself it was what I needed to do to be desirable. At the gay circuit parties, it was all about the hookup with gorgeous men, it was all about the sex. Not about relationships. These guys were not enthralled by my intellect or wit. They just wanted to use the body I presented them to get off, and then move on to the next one. I had been a willing participant for far too long, and it was time to stop. It was time to find my center and roll the dice to see whether the true Brandon beneath all the trauma was worth loving. Worth saving. I was ready to take that next step toward wholeness.

I sat with CeCe's question, and decided it was time to take off the suit and put it away.

"Okay, in those 10 years, was there ever a time when you looked in the mirror and said 'wow. I finally look the way I've wanted to look?'"

I replied with one word. "No."

CeCe smiled and said, "Great! You've done it your way for ten years and you still aren't happy with your body. Now, it's my turn. You're going to do it my way from this point on. Flush all the steroids down the drain. No more injections. No more 3000-calorie shakes."

I could do this. I had to do it. I did as she instructed. I was ready.

"Every morning, I want you look at yourself in the mirror and repeat the following ten times in a row. 'You are enough.'

"Are you kidding? You really think that will change anything?"

She knew me better than I did myself in some ways. I hated looking at myself in the mirror. I hated taking pictures because I hated what I looked like. I know you're thinking that makes no sense because I make my living speaking in front of a camera in front of tens of thousands of people every night. I had spent my whole life looking in the mirror or at a picture and had repeated one phrase, if only in my mind, millions of times. "I hate what I look like." That lead to self-loathing and self-harm. She was helping me change the script, and so I did as she told me.

I trusted her. Her strategy was simple: strip me of all the outside noise and down to the bare basics. She was teaching me to love myself the way God made me. This sounds so basic, but standing in front of the mirror and saying "You are enough" over and over again actually started to work. Without the steroids and super shakes, I dropped 40 pounds.

About a year later, the miracle that I had been praying for most of my life occurred. I stood in front of my mirror naked and I looked at my body. I was now 166 pounds. I was me again, and I smiled. For the first time in my entire life, I liked the reflection in the mirror. I cried. Tears streamed down my face. I screamed "Holy shit, it worked! Positive affirmation actually worked!"

My hate affair turned into a love affair. I was being kind to myself and I no longer had negative thoughts running through my mind while looking into the mirror. I had never trusted that anyone would be attracted to me. I was killing myself attracting the wrong people for the wrong reasons. But I began receiving more attention from guys at 165 pounds than I did all juiced up at 205. The biggest difference was that these were not the chiseled gladiators that I had once convinced myself I could not live without.

The gay circuit world is dangerous. It bends your perceptions and makes you feel like you're inadequate. Makes you feel like you're not good enough. Why else would 99% of the guys who go to circuit parties take so many drugs and inject themselves with so many steroids? From my experience, they do it to get attention. They do it because they are not happy with their natural selves.

I know many gay men who are reading this book right now – who are part of the circuit world – are cursing at me. I'm not saying this to shame the guys in that circuit world. Heck, do whatever you want with your body and life. I only want to shed light on the fact there is another reality in which you are perfect just the way you are. It does not exist in the sex and drug parties.

Many of you are like I was, hurting deep inside. It is like this hole, this void that can never be filled and can never be satisfied. You are starving all the time, and yet nothing fills you. The circuit parties are nothing but smoke and funhouse mirrors that distort the truth, and because you are vulnerable and maybe under the influence of drugs and alcohol, you believe the image you are witnessing is real. It's a lie.

I call those lost in this diabolical world The Lost Boys. I started partying in the circuit scene when I was 19. Taking drugs to party half-naked on the dance floor looking like incredible Hulk is not normal. I know many men in that world who are trapped. They feel like if they quit, they would never laugh again or be desired. They believe their life will be boring and meaningless.

I truly felt I would never have fun again when I left the circuit scene. The truth is, I have more fun sober than I did at any of those circuit parties. I have never laughed so hard. I am able to feel and connect with other human beings on such a deeper level now. I could never do that in my old life.

AA FOR NORMIES

I've said it once and I'll say it a million times over: The 12 Steps in AA aren't just proven to have a positive impact in the lives of addicts. People who are not addicts—we in AA call them "Normies"—can also improve the quality of their lives by working some of the steps. Below are some of the 12 steps and examples how each can help you navigate through a life struggle. I have bolded the word alcohol, because you can substitute whatever word you would like that represents a struggle you may be having in your life.

1) *We admitted we were powerless over **alcohol** - that our lives had become unimaginable.*

Try replacing the word alcohol and replace it with the word sex. It works, right? Now try replacing it with words like food, smoking, swearing, video games, etc. You will instantly see that a vast majority of Americans qualify to work the 12 Steps.

2) *Come to believe that a power greater than ourselves could restore us to sanity.*

This really doesn't need much of an explanation other than admitting you are not the most powerful person in the world. Unless, of course, you're a world leader and are clinically narcissistic.

3) *You've made a decision to turn our will and our lives over to the care of God as we understood him.*

Essentially you are letting go of things that are out of your control and giving them to someone else. Another exercise I like to do is something called a God Box that lives under my bed. I write down things that are bothering me. Things I have no control over or can't seem to find a solution to. I write it down on a piece of paper, say a prayer about it, and then I place that paper into that God Box (a shoe box) and close the lid and don't think about it again. When I do think about it, I remind myself I already handed it off to someone else.

4) *You've made a searching and fearless moral inventory of yourself.*

This is by far the most crucial step to improving our lives. Not just as addicts, but as people. We all have examples in our lives of events that transpired because our moral compass went south. We've all done things we are not proud of. Things that we often bury in a closet and purposely lose the key so that no one will ever find out about them. The problem with that is, your closet will eventually overflow, and all that shit will hit the next person who tries to crack the door open to your soul. In essence, clean your dirty laundry by doing the step work. You will experience healthier relationships down the road.

5) *Admit to God, to ourselves, and to another human being the exact nature of our wrongs*

You know that saying, "I feel the weight of the world on my shoulders." This step allows us to tell someone, even through prayer, what we did wrong that day. Just by telling someone else, and not keeping that buried in our souls, takes away some of the power it has over us. We all mess up. Every single day. No one is perfect. We may lie, exaggerate, forge a document, yell at a phone operator about a billing issue. Whatever it is, we need to tell someone so that it doesn't consume us and lead us back to that behavior we admitted in the first step.

6) *We were entirely ready to have God remove all these defects of character.*

We all have character defects. Stop trying to portray a perfect life, in reality or on social media. It's disingenuous. It's not relatable. Why do you think most people never get sick of listening to Oprah? She's everywhere. TV, magazines, etc. Yet, she still has more followers than any other human being and her likeability score is off the charts decade after decade. It's because she's authentic and she has shown all of us her character defects. It makes her relatable. Like her struggle with weight loss. Because she's brave enough to show us her scars, we relate.

7) *Humbly ask Him to remove our shortcomings.*

We are imperfect beings, blessed and cursed with free will. We have the free will to really screw up our lives and negatively impact those around us. Isn't it nice that we can have someone help us not only clean up our mess but also to help us stop repeating the actions that brought on the mess to begin with? We don't have to go about our lives alone. We are never alone, and He always has our back.

We ask for help, and do it humbly. We accept our shortcomings, acknowledge them, and ask for help. We do it without ego and without any other agenda than to become the best version of ourselves.

8) *Make a list of all persons we had harmed and became willing to make amends to them all.*

If Step 4 is the most important, then steps 8 and 9 are tied for a close second. If we are to become better people, we have to admit when we are wrong. It's humbling. It's not easy to admit we fucked up (especially if no one saw us do it!). But we all hurt other people, knowingly or by accident. We must apologize. If we don't, then people will not want to work with us, be friends with us, or be married to us. We become that asshole no one likes.

Don't ever listen to people who say, "never apologize" or "never admit wrongdoing." That is the worst advice I have ever heard, and I cringe when I see politicians use that same tactic. Imagine if we had a president who said, "I owe the American people an apology. I was mistaken when I promised you this. I was wrong, and I hope we can forge together through compromise a way to make it right". Holy shit. That president just might get an approval rating above 50%!

9) *Make direct amends to such people wherever possible,*
except when to do so would injure them or others.

Remember, when we make amends to people in our lives whom we have wronged, we never point out their character defects or their wrongdoings. We apologize only for our behavior. When you do that, you will be surprised at how others react. In my experience, when I apologize for my behavior in an incident, the other person usually follows with an apology. It's like a domino effect of accountability.

10) *Continue to take personal inventory and when*
we were wrong promptly admitted it.

This should be done nightly, before resting our heads on our pillows. You can do this with a pen and paper or just speak out loud. We think about what happened that day and we ask ourselves: Did we do anything that we need to apologize for? If so, we do it immediately. If we don't act promptly, we really are risking everything, and it will likely lead us back to our vices.

11) *Sought through prayer and meditation to improve our conscious*
contact with God, as we understood Him, praying only for knowledge
of His will for us and the power to carry that out.

Meditating has been one of the biggest challenges for me. I can't seem to sit still for longer than five minutes without my mind racing into a billion different directions. But prayer works for me.

I only pray for a few minutes. It's hard to describe in words, but try it and I guarantee you, you will see results. This step is also important in that we don't pray for specifics: I pray for a bigger salary, etc. This is about praying to understand what God's will for me. We all have a purpose here on Earth. Sorry, it's not to win the lottery, live in a mansion, be a supermodel, or drive a Porsche. Simply ask, "God, just guide me in the right direction. Make the path obvious for me to follow. I pray that you keep me in good health. Put me wherever anyone needs to hear a message of hope."

12) *Having had that spiritual awakening as the result of these steps, we tried to carry this message to alcoholics, and to practice these principles in all our affairs.*

In AA, we work with other addicts to get them sober. In return, we get to stay sober. For all my Normies reading his book, this step is about service work. What are you doing for your community to make it better? What actions are you taking that are selfless? Are you volunteering for a charitable group? Did you take a few minutes to say hello to a stranger? Did you pause and ask someone at work genuinely how they're doing? It's about giving back FIRST, before expecting anything in return. Essentially, if you want good karma coming your way, you better learn to be nice and do for others without expecting them to return the goodwill.

8

The Crooked Way Home

I don't want to appear ungrateful or give the impression that AA, NA, and CMA are not great organizations that have helped people, including me, to become sober. But I believe there are a number of aspects about these organizations that are not healthy and are not often addressed publicly. One of them is the anonymous component; we just are not supposed to talk about it. There is also an emotional component that the journey of sobriety is a tough one and so it seems crass to say anything disparaging about the teachings or the meetings.

While AA/NA/CMA works well for many, many people, it is not the only pathway to sobriety. There are many paths, and one is not any more valid than the other if it works for the individual. The problem is when the attitude within the protective halls of AA rooms is one of judgement, fear, and superiority.

I still consider myself a member of AA, and a success story, but there is a lingering, embedded amount of fear and shame when I decided to take a break from attending meetings for a few months. I needed a break to allow some growth and I increased the frequency of my therapy sessions. The response I received from my brothers and sisters in AA was not positive. In fact, it was downright nasty.

GAY AA/NA/CMA MEETINGS

The premise is sound. Having a safe place for gay people to meet and share their stories makes sense. There are a number of gay-only AA clubhouses around the country. To me, at times it felt anything but safe and inviting.

Before and after the meetings, guys would come up and hug me and tell me they were glad to see me, and for the most part these were genuine and innocent. But there were several men who took a different approach. They would grab my ass. Touch me inappropriately. And say things to me that made me feel dirty and sexualized. Some guys even had the nerve to try to kiss me on the lips.

This was not the safe brotherhood that I needed. This happened often in the gay AA meetings I attended in Atlanta. The problem is that these meetings made it all right to act this way. They felt entitled to act inappropriately, because they were not seeing it as inappropriate. It was accepted, and all part of being in gay AA together. I did not agree! I was looking for chances to leave the meetings early so that I would not be approached and groped afterwards. It got so bad that I discussed my experiences with my sponsor at the time, CeCe, and she agreed I needed to find a different meeting to attend.

I could not quit AA because I had to go. I was still early in my sobriety, and I needed the meetings. "Meeting Makers Make It!" is one of the sayings plastered on every wall of every AA meeting hall. I decided to begin attending straight AA meetings instead. I felt much safer in those meetings because I was not approached or harassed.

Then I decided to take a break. After going to meetings for so long, they became a bit monotonous. Some of the people in these meetings have been coming for twenty years. They are still bitching about the same things and the same people. It is draining when you have to sit, smile, and applaud their feigned courage week after week. I was becoming jaded and needed a break.

I talked it over with my therapist, and she agreed that a break would be fine as long as we met more often. I was trying to figure out what the next part of my life journey was going to be. I was gaining more insight and support from my therapist than from the meetings. But inside, there was this nagging feeling. This thought that if I did not go, I would relapse. Once an addict, always an addict. It is like this terminal disease that you can never shake. If I did not take my prescribed AA medicine, I could relapse and die.

One morning after a rigorous tennis match, I went to one of my favorite breakfast joints. As I walked in I saw my regular AA home group of men sitting together. They spotted me as I spotted them. I would have expected that they would have given me a warm, "Hey, Brandon, it is so great to see you! How are you doing?"

Oh no... I got glares. I got the eyes rolling from my head to my feet and back again, with a flourishing eye roll to accent their disapproval.

"Hey, Brandon. Where have you been? You have not been to meetings lately. Are you still sober?"

I felt burning in my cheeks. The audacity of their judgement was like a stinging slap to my face. It is not uncommon for people in AA to feel superior, pure, and godly. Some gay men are the worst in that department. They triggered doubt, insecurity, and shame that I was not attending, but I refused to show that they had hit a nerve.

"Yes, I am sober and loving life. I am doing fantastic. I just finished a great tennis match, I'm here to refuel, and life is great. How are you guys?"

I had to process this feeling it had left me. I was not working the AA plan, so was I destined to relapse and taking a train straight to hell? How could they judge me in such a way? How could they make me feel so despised, like I was some failure?

"Why does that bother you so much?" my therapist asked.

"I have this feeling of shame and guilt. It has been ingrained into me from these 12 Step programs. I am an addict. I am an alcoholic. Because I have decided to take a break, I am risking everything," I replied.

"Stop labeling yourself, Brandon. You are not a drug addict anymore. You are a changed man. You have done the work. You are labelling yourself something so negative that does not apply to who you are now."

At first, I challenged her. Once an addict, always an addict. But then I began to see the light. That was not me anymore. I was not the man I was nine years ago. I had fundamentally changed my entire life. I no longer desired to drink or do drugs. Why did I need to carry that burden and label? It is something I continue to work through, but I don't think the fear aspect that AA preaches has helped my sobriety or my self-esteem in these later years into recovery.

I still consider myself a member of AA; after all, the only requirement to join is having a desire to stop drinking. That's it. I travel the country sharing my story. I speak at AA conventions and share a story of hope and inspiration to other addicts who are desperate to hear success stories. I am excited about an upcoming opportunity to speak at a convention during World Pride in New York City in the summer of 2019. The more I speak at conventions, the more I get asked to share my story in other cities. This is what I believe my life calling is: sharing my story of addiction with others who are suffering. But, as your about to read, not everyone is so willing to hear a message of hope.

A MAN WITH AN AX TO GRIND

After a certain number of years of being sober, it is natural for a person in AA to become a sponsor for someone early in their sobriety. I have had multiple sponsees, even a few at a time. We meet weekly, usually on Sunday, and we do exercises from the AA Big Book and talk through their issues. I am there for them whenever they need me. If they feel they are going to relapse, I talk them through the challenges they are facing and the possible consequences should they slip.

I guide my sponsees through the 12 steps and work toward their first year of sobriety. Because what we talk about is personal, it has been normal for me in the past to invite my sponsees to my house. It is a much quieter and safer place than a coffee house. At least, I thought it was safe.

While I was living and working in Atlanta, I observed a crystal meth addict, let's call him Tom, coming in and out of the Crystal Meth Anonymous group for a year or two. He would be sober for a few months and attend regularly, and then he would relapse and disappear for a time.

I was celebrating one of my AA birthdays—a certain number of years being sober—when Tom approached me. He asked if I would be his sponsor, and my heart sank. I wanted to say no, but I was taught that while in sobriety, you never say no to service work. My reluctance to working with Tom was that I was not sure I could help him. I had seen his patterns of addiction, and I was afraid I would not be effective to someone who did not seem ready to commit to sobriety.

I said yes, and we began working together for a couple of months. Everything seemed to go well. He came to my house with my other sponsees and he seemed to be doing the work. Then suddenly, he vanished for a week. I did not hear anything from him, and I figured that he relapsed again.

At this time, I was working as a morning anchor for the CBS affiliate in Atlanta. This meant my day started early. I woke up at 1:00 am and left my house about 2 am. Because of the early mornings, I wanted to be able to pull out of my garage going forward, and so every evening I backed my truck in.

I started my truck as I always did. I hit the remote to open the garage and waited for it to open. This one morning there was something waiting for me on the other side.

The garage door inched upwards and in my headlights I saw in my driveway a pair of shoes.

Then I saw a pair of legs.

Then I saw a waist.

Then, an ax.

My stomach dropped. Oh, my God. Who the fuck was standing in my driveway holding an ax?

The garage door continued to open. I saw his arms, then his chest, and then his neck. Finally his face was revealed. I froze in terror. It was Tom. His eyes were bugged out. They were huge. It looked as though he was on something like bath salts or meth.

Once his eyes locked with mine, he began screaming at me.

"Tom, what are you doing here?" I asked.

"They are trying to kill me. You are trying to kill me. I am going to fucking kill you."

None of it was making sense, and I panicked. I began screaming loudly, more like high-pitched squealing. My first impulse was to close the garage, as if that would stop a homicidal killer with an ax. I pressed the button. Just as slowly as it had crept up, it began to close, chain link by chain link. I sat frozen in terror in my front seat, not sure what to do next. Once the garage door closed, I grabbed my phone.

"This is 911, what is your emergency?" a voice on the line said.

"There is a guy in my driveway. I know who he is. He is a drug addict. I am pretty sure he is high on drugs now. He has an ax and he is going to kill me."

I went back into my house to wait for the police. I hoped Tom would not decide to use the ax to break into my house. I went to my bedroom when I heard a crash. I looked out toward Tom's place. He lived only two apartment buildings away, and I could view his apartment from mine. He had pushed his large window air conditioner from his window in order to escape whomever he thought was coming after him.

The police arrived quickly and arrested him. Once they took my statement, I went to work. I was very shaken, but I tried to put the whole terrifying incident behind me.

Two weeks later I was sitting in a CMA meeting when in walked Tom. He walked over and sat down next to me with a smile. I was in shock. I did not know what to say or do.

"Hey, man, how are you?" he asked. Still with the same smile, as if everything was perfectly normal.

"I'm fine" is all I could really say at first. "Um . . . do you even remember what happened?"

By his demeanor, I did not think that he remembered, which was not totally out of the realm of possibility, as I myself had blacked out a number of times while under the influence of drugs.

"What are you talking about?" Tom asked.

I could have just let it go, especially he had no memory of what he had done. But I couldn't. He had to be made aware of what he had done to me. He needed to be given the chance to apologize and make amends. Also, I was pissed.

"Do you remember what happened two weeks ago? Let's take this outside for a chat."

He followed me outside the meeting room. His face looked worried.

"What's going on, man?" he asked in a defensive tone.

"Dude. Two weeks ago you showed up at 2:00 am at my house with an ax in your hand. You threatened to kill me."

I could see confusion cross his expression. "Oh, my God. Were you the person that called the cops on me?"

This did not feel like an apology and so my temper took over.

"Absolutely I did. You had a fucking ax. You looked at me like Michael Myers from Halloween intent on killing me. In fact, you were screaming at me that was what you wanted to do."

"I am so sorry. I relapsed. I was high on drugs and I was hallucinating. I thought people were after me. I thought you were after me."

I explained that because I did not feel safe with him, I could no longer be his sponsor. I would continue to be supportive of his sobriety during the meetings, but I could not offer him anything further.

Because of being anonymous, I never knew his last name, and so I am not sure what ever happened to Tom. I hope he eventually found his way.

The thing about crystal meth addicts is that the drug will keep you awake for days. After a couple of days of not having sleep, the person will become paranoid. Peeking through the curtains, *they are coming to get me* level paranoid.

Step 12 of AA is help others. It is at this point you can become a sponsor. The idea of being a sponsor is that it gives your life purpose and therefore helps you remain sober. During my celebration of going through all the steps, a person named John approached me to be his sponsor. My sponsor, CeCe, was standing next to me and said, "Brandon would be happy to be your sponsor."

I was not so sure, but she reminded me of my commitment and that I needed to do it. John was similar to Tom in that he was a crystal meth addict who would be on and off sober for 30 days at a time. I worked hard with John, and he made it to a year of sobriety. Then, like Tom, he vanished and relapsed.

He called me. "Man, I need your help, Brandon. I am in a bad place."

"When was the last time you used?" I knew his drug of choice was meth, and I remembered my experience with Tom.

"About two days ago."

"I make it rule not to visit until it has been 72 hours since your last use. I will talk to you tomorrow."

I went to his apartment the next day, and he was looking through the windows, still trapped by the drug and lack of sleep. He was absolutely convinced someone was coming for him. Even when I explained it was the meth that was making him paranoid, and that there was no one coming for him, he would not believe me.

After working as a sponsor for a number of addicts, I became despondent. Most of my sponsees had relapsed. I approached CeCe and asked her what I was doing wrong.

"Have you relapsed?" she asked me.

"No," I replied.

"Then your success rate is 100%. Being a sponsor is not about them as much as it is about you, Brandon. It is to help you continue your sobriety, not to be a savior. They have their work, just as you had yours. The fact you are still sober is a success. Remember that."

No one ever said getting sober was easy. No one ever told me how my moral compass would be tested within the rooms of AA. It's so important people understand this: just because someone is in AA getting sober does not mean they are trustworthy or honest or even a good person. A lot of people in AA have committed terrible crimes against others. Addicts are liars, cheaters, thieves, and manipulators. The list goes on and on. I didn't learn this until I started working with others trying to get them clean.

I like to try new AA meetings from time to time to keep it fresh. I shared my story at a new AA clubhouse in Atlanta. I had about four years of sobriety at the time. A man who appeared homeless came up to me after the meeting and asked me to be his sponsor. Remember, in AA, we are taught to never say no to service work. Never say no to helping another addict trying to get sober. But my gut was telling me this guy was trouble. Something about him seemed off.

I did what I was taught and I agreed to work with him. At our first meeting he said, "Brandon, I have something to share with you, but I'm scared."

I told him he could share anything he wanted with me and that it would be totally confidential. He didn't feel comfortable with me yet and I totally understood. A few one-on-one meetings later, he finally shared his big dark secret.

"Brandon, I have been doing something terrible."

Now, up to this point I thought I'd heard it all. Nothing could shock me. Nothing could scare me off. I said, "What's going on? You can share it with me. If you don't then the pain will live inside your soul and you will eventually pick up a drink over it. But if you tell me, you will take its power away."

I don't even remember his name. In AA we never ask people for their last name. After all, it is Alcoholics Anonymous.

His head was bowed. He was staring at the floor. I told him to look up and look me in the eyes. He did and that's when he dropped a bombshell I wasn't prepared to handle.

"Brandon, I have done something so terrible. I have been raping my girlfriends seven-year-old daughter."

Holy shit. I tried not to look panicked. I wanted him to tell me more. I wanted him to keep sharing. I had earned his trust.

I asked him, "What have you been doing to this little girl?"

He said, "I've been kissing her on the couch when her mom isn't home. I'm homeless, so I've been staying with this girl and it's her daughter. I have penetrated her twice."

My heart was racing. I was full of rage. I wanted to beat the living shit out of this guy. I kept my cool. It was almost like an out-of-body experience.

I asked him, "When was the last time this happened?"

He said, "Last night."

My palms were sweaty. I had sweat beads dripping down my back. I wasn't taught how to handle this. I was taught to keep everything a secret between me and my sponsees. I was told never ever to betray that trust. What was I supposed to do? I couldn't NOT say anything. I had to do something. So I told a confidant of mine in AA. I told him what my sponsee told me. This confidant didn't know who my sponsee was and so I wasn't breaking his trust. I need advice and I needed it quick.

My confidant told me, "Brandon, don't say anything. You can't betray his trust. You would be wrong to tell anyone, and you shouldn't even be telling me!"

I was shaking at this point. I called my sponsor CeCe. I told her everything my homeless sponsee confessed to me. This was happening in real time, too. My sponsee who just admitted he was raping a 7-year-old girl was inside the AA clubhouse. I told him I had to step outside to take a phone call.

CeCe replied, "Brandon, you MUST go to police."

I felt better. I called my best friend Hannah. She too said "B, you have to go to police right now."

My next call was to a detective with the Atlanta PD. She

asked me for his name.

"Shit. I don't know his last name. It's AA. We don't tell people our last names."

The detective came up with a plan. She wanted to trick my sponsee into giving us his real name so cops could identify him and arrest him for suspicion of child rape.

"Brandon. Here's what you're going to do. You're going to ask him if he needs help finding a job. Tell him that you have connections that can get him work immediately. But you're going to tell him that in order for you to help him, he will need to provide you with a copy of his identification or driver's license."

Sure enough, the guy gave me a copy of his ID and I immediately sent it to the cop. The detective said "OK. Good job Brandon. We're almost there. I know this is not easy for you, but you are doing the right thing. If you hadn't said anything, you'd be considered an accomplice. One more thing I need from you. I need him to tell you where his girlfriend lives. I need to know where he's staying and where the abuse is happening."

I went back inside the clubhouse. I asked my sponsee, "Hey, do you need a lift back to your girlfriend's house? I can take you there, so you won't have to take the bus."

"No. I'm OK. I'll take the bus."

Shoot. What do I do now? I insisted. But he got spooked. Something set him off and he literally took off running. I didn't even have his phone number. I called the detective back and said,

"He wouldn't let me take him home. I don't know where the girlfriend lives."

The detective said "That's OK, Brandon. You have done the right thing. I know this isn't easy, but you are trying to protect the little girl."

I too was a victim of child sex abuse. I was molested multiple times as a child. How could I possibly live with myself or even sleep at night knowing that a man was raping an innocent little girl. And what mother would ever invite a homeless man into her house and then leave the child unattended with them?

I've shared this story in AA meetings and I have to be honest with you, the reaction has been mixed. I have had people come up to me saying that I handled it all wrong. Some say I shouldn't have said anything. Some people hugged me and told me I did the right thing. This was the beginning of my resentment toward AA and the rooms of AA. Our first priority shouldn't be to protect someone at all costs just because they're in the rooms of AA. Hell, no. Our first priority should always be the victims. Always. At the end of each AA meetings we say this prayer: "God, grant me the serenity to accept the things I cannot change, the courage to change the things I can, and the wisdom to know the difference. God, we pray for those who are suffering inside these rooms..." I began to add this line to that prayer and I say it out loud, "And Lord, we ask that you protect the children who don't have a say in the matter."

Children are powerless. They can't stop their parents from drinking. They are innocent victims. Period. We must always do what we can to protect them even if that means going against the AA principles.

The detective called me about a week later and said they hadn't been able to track him down. My heart sank. I don't know where that man is today either. I never saw him at that meeting again. I even went to more meetings than usual hoping to find him. I would have done a citizen's arrest if I saw him. Looking back, I wish I had the courage to tackle him to the ground and hold him there until cops got there. There isn't a week that goes by that I don't think about some innocent little girl being raped. I feel at times that I failed that little girl and it hurts my heart and brings tears to my eyes. Even all these years later.

FINDING HOPE IN PRISON

When I first walked into the rooms of AA, I had no idea what to expect. I'd never heard of the famous 12 Steps. I didn't know what would happen or how my life would change as drastically as it has ... for the better.

We've talked about the importance of the 12th step:

Having had a spiritual awakening as the result of these

steps, we try to carry this message to alcoholics, and to
practice these principles in all our affairs.

When we first get sober, the only person we think about is ourselves. We have a saying in AA that it's a selfish program. It has to be. If an addict doesn't focus solely on themselves and change their behavior and rewire their brains, then the addict is of no use to anyone else. How can I be a good friend, brother, son, husband if I can't string together time in sobriety? Once we get through the first 11 steps, we then begin the 12th step. It's the step that keeps me sober. I can only maintain my sobriety if I pass on my experience to another addict who is suffering.

When I moved to Phoenix, I didn't know a single person. The first thing I did was hit a meeting when I got there. I went to a place called Crossroads. It's a place that houses newly sober addicts. It also hosts some of the best AA meetings in all of Phoenix. There are people with 24 hours of sobriety and people who are 50 years sober. One night I was asked to share my story in front of the group. I had about five years sober at the time. I shared my story briefly before we broke out in discussion groups. Immediately after I spoke, this young guy, Zach (not his real name), came up to me and asked me to be his sponsor. He pulled me aside and told me about himself. He was newly sober and his drug of choice was heroin. He had just gotten out of prison for theft and drug possession. The courts sent him to AA meetings.

Now, most of my normie friends said, "Brandon, why the hell are you spending time with a guy who robs people and shoots heroin? Are you fucking crazy?"

I know it sounds crazy to the outside world, but I have no fear working with another alcoholic, even those who've committed violent crimes (except when they show up in my driveway with an ax.) And trust me, there are a lot of people with rap sheets in AA. But people change. I've seen it not only in myself, but in so many others. I have watched people's lives transform right in front of my eyes. It's a beautiful thing to see a hopeless soul grow into a bright, shining example of good.

Zach asked me to be his sponsor, which meant I would work with him several days a week going through the steps. It's a grueling process but it's one that is so rewarding. It's almost hard to put into words when you see someone get clean.

He had ruined many relationships in his life. His parents were on the verge of disowning him. He'd used his parents too many times for money and housing and he kept fucking it all up. He was rude, disrespectful, the list goes on. He said to me at our first meeting, "Brandon, I have to get clean, man. I have to change. I don't want to go back to prison."

I told him if he did what I tell him to do, then he'd avoid prison and his life would eventually come together, and he'd be able to amend the relationships in his life that had soured.

Zach was doing great. He never missed a meeting with me.

He did all the assignments I gave him. He never complained. He got a job. He made enough money to pay his own rent without calling mom for money. Just that simple change in behavior was the beginning of the rebuilding process in that important relationship with mom and son.

I told him, "Zach if you focus on you and only you, everyone else will see the beautiful change in you and they will want to be part of your life. You don't have to force it."

Before he knew it, he earned his one year sobriety chip. Never before had he reached an entire year without a drink or a drug. Then, all of a sudden, he didn't show up to meet me for step work and coffee.

I thought to myself, "Well, that's strange. He never misses a meeting with me and he's not answering his phone." I called and texted one time each. That's it. I do not chase down my sponsees. Ever. They are grown men. If they want to get wasted and screw up their life, that's their decision and it has no impact on me. Disappointing, sure. But, as cruel as this may sound, "better him than me." Remember, the reason why I work with so many sponsees in the program is because it keeps me sober. I get the gift of sobriety when I give the gift of sobriety. It's that simple.

About six months went by and I never heard from Zach. Then, one day, my phone rang. I didn't recognize the number and I usually send those calls straight to voicemail. But for some reason I answered, not knowing who was on the other line. I am so grateful I answered. It wasn't Zach; it was his mother.

She said to me, "Brandon, I need your help. Zach's in trouble. He's in jail right now. He's facing 25 years to life. He begged me to call you. He has a sentencing date next week and we'd really like for you to speak on his behalf in front of the judge with the hope of getting a reduced sentence. But it's not looking good at all right now."

Another lesson I've learned in recovery is when another addict needs help, we don't hesitate. We go. We do.

I showed up for court and there he was dressed in his orange jumpsuit with his inmate number plastered across his chest. He looked like the shell of the man I was working with. He looked like he'd been on a bender. He looked like shit. But when he turned his head over to us in the courtroom, we made eye contact. He smiled for a brief moment, and then he broke down crying. This is the power of an addict looking another addict in the eyes. You cannot bullshit another addict. He was so ashamed of what he did.

I had warned him multiple times while working with him that he shouldn't date or have sex for a year. He didn't want to follow that rule. Sure enough, he got hooked up with a girl who happened to be a drug runner for a cartel in Arizona. According to him, he was staying at her house when she was sick. She was apparently so sick she couldn't make a drug delivery. In the cartel world, if you fail to make a delivery, they will assume you stole the drugs and they'll kill you.

Zach decided to help his girlfriend. He chose to deliver the drugs for her. He walked out of her house to make the delivery to the car outside. The guys got out. Turns out it wasn't another drug dealer, it was the FBI. Game over.

Zach was locked up immediately. They didn't care to listen to his story. Why should they? He had a rap sheet.

It was my turn to walk up to the microphone inside the courtroom. You could hear a pin drop. My heart was racing. I don't like courtrooms. I also knew Zach's life was in jeopardy.

"Your honor. My name is Brandon Lee. I have five years sober. I'm a news anchor here in Phoenix. I am someone who was once addicted to drugs, but the AA program has turned my life around. I met Zach at an AA meeting and he asked me to be his sponsor. I worked him daily. I took him through all 12 steps. He had a job. He was paying his own rent. I watched him rebuild relationships with his family. I've watched him get promoted to manager of the halfway house he was living in. I have even watched him help new addicts get sober. I'm not sure why Zach stopped calling me, but I believe we all know why now. I'm not here to make excuses for Zach.

"I am here simply to say that I have seen Zach at his worst and I've seen him at his best. When he commits to a life of sobriety, he has the ability to contribute to our society. Down deep he is a compassionate young man who had a rough childhood. Prison is no place for an addict. He won't get better in a jail cell. He needs sobriety. He needs to be around other sober people. Your honor, I ask that you do not sentence him to life in prison. I'm also not asking that he go unpunished. He must pay back his debts to society for what he's done. But I also know that unless he gets treatment, this pattern of behavior will never end."

The judge called for a recess to think about the sentence in his chambers. When he came back into the courtroom, everyone stood up. The judge looked at Zach and said, "I hope you understand how many people love you. These people have taken time out of their day to be here to speak on your behalf. Your sponsor makes a few good points. Prison is not a place for drug addicts. You need help. But I can't let you go unpunished. I am sentencing you to two years in prison, and then you will enter a recovery program when you're released."

Zach broke down crying. He thought his life was over, but he'd been given another chance. I haven't spoken to Zach since I saw him in the courtroom that day. I may never see or talk with him again. But I was there for him, just as the AA program taught me to be.

His mother has reached out multiple times to thank me. She even said Zach is holding AA meetings in prison! She says he recommitted to the program of recovery. That tells me to never give up hope on an addict. You don't have to give them money or limitless emotional support. Some addicts get the message. Other addicts are the message. Not everyone gets sober. It's sad but true.

People have to figure it out on their own time table. I've seen people hit rock bottom, only to watch them fall deeper when I didn't think it could get any worse for them.

BREAKING DOWN

There was no linear, easy path to follow with my sex addiction. In some ways it was harder than beating drug addiction because sex is a natural part of life, not something you just stop doing forever. I had to learn to shift my mindset about sex and about relationships. But, as they say, habits die hard.

In 2010, when I started with my first sponsor, Joel, he had a lot of rules. I mean, a lot of rules. No sex. No porn. No dating. What kind of life is that? He told me from the beginning he would only work with me if I was willing to do anything and everything to get sober. I said yes, so I couldn't question him. In addition to those rules, he had me call him every single day for the first year. No texting. I had to pick up the phone, dial his number, let it ring, and actually speak to him on the phone. Even if nothing was happening, I still had to check in with him. I have never called anyone every day. Never. Not friends. Not my family. No one. I was accountable only to myself.

I obliged. I called him every single day. Sometimes it was quick, "Hey it's me. All good here! Bye!"

I was about 6 months sober at the time and I was working the program just as my sponsor had directed me. We met face to face every weekend. We read the Big Book together. We did written exercises. I was praying morning and night. I was an A student in AA. One thing I will likely always be: an overachiever.

I was driving down Peachtree Road in Atlanta one Saturday afternoon. Everything was fine. I was in a good place emotionally. I was excited about a dinner party with friends that night. As I was driving I saw out of the corner of my eye a sign that read FLEX. I did a double take. My heart was racing. Butterflies in my stomach. Before I knew it, my hands turned the steering wheel to the left, cutting across four lanes of traffic nearly crashing into multiple cars.

I pulled into the parking lot and sure enough, it was the same fucking bathhouse where I used to get high and have sex for days. Only this time, I wasn't in LA, I was in Atlanta. You mean to tell me this bathhouse is a fucking chain? Like a fast food restaurant?

I sat in the parking lot for a solid 20 minutes. I was hypnotized watching anonymous men walk in and out of the bathhouse, eerily similar to the scene in LA. Guys carrying backpacks that I knew were filled with drugs. I told myself, "Brandon, you can do this. You can go inside and have sex and not do any drugs. You can do this! Come on, man!"

That was the devil on my shoulder. He never went away. He was doing pushups, getting stronger, waiting for me to have a weak moment. This was the devil's chance to get me to relapse.

I didn't have a crack pipe in my car. I'm sober now. So that instinct to look in my center console turned up nothing. Instead I ended up grabbing my cell phone. I looked at it, and something came over me and took control. I started dialing my sponsor's phone number.

"Hey, Brandon, how are you?"

"Joel. I'm sitting in a parking lot of a bathhouse on Peachtree Road. FLEX. The same bathhouse I used to get loaded at."

Joel was calm on the other end. "OK. Why are you there?" he asked.

"I don't know. I was driving down the road and I saw the sign in the corner of my eye, and I ended up in the parking lot," I replied.

"OK. What's happening right now?" he asked in a calm voice.

"Well, I'm watching these guys go in and out. They all look high on drugs."

"Brandon. Just do what I tell you to do, OK? Put your keys in the ignition. Start your car. Put the car in drive."

I did as he said. Still in a zombie-like state of mind. Joel heard my car start and said, "Brandon, I am going to stay on the phone with you, OK? I need you to put the car in drive and get out of there now."

I did as he instructed. The moment my car left the parking lot, I started breathing heavily. The weight lifted. I was so relieved.

I started crying in joy. I knew I had just escaped a relapse. I beat the devil that day and it's only because I did what my sponsor had asked. He got me to call him every day. Not because he wanted to hear from me; rather, he was training me for that exact moment. Because I called him every day anyway, the phone didn't feel like a 50-pound weight. I just called him naturally.

Sometimes I like to question authority and make them explain to me why they're having me do something. But I never questioned Joel about calling. Did I like it? Hell no! I hated calling him daily. But it was another life lesson: sometimes we need to do what we're told because someone else knows better. I was willing to do anything and everything to stay sober.

Me: 1

Devil: 0

MONDAY MOTIVATIONS

Again, I don't want to seem like I am not appreciative of AA/NA/CMA, because frankly it saved my life. Like any huge organization it has its issues, but they do help people when they are ready to give their lives over to something bigger than themselves.

A few years ago I started a Facebook thread called Monday Motivations. I posted quotes from a book called Daily Reflections. While it's endorsed by AA, anyone could find wisdom within its pages. Along with the daily reflection, I would post my feelings about it. It was the first time I came out publicly that I was a recovering drug addict. It was a bit of testing of the waters. I had to be authentic about my addiction to give my responses context. I did not know what to expect.

As people read them they began responding to me in private. There was no shame or guilt, only support and confirmation that I was not alone. People shared their own addiction stories, both personal and about friends and family members. This was significant to me and one of the reasons I decided to write this book. I have spoken at AA conferences all around the country, but I had never stepped beyond the walls of recovery to share my message. Because of the positive outpouring of support, I knew it was time to spread my message of hope further.

HEALTHY OUTLETS

As an addict, I admit I had a lot of vices. Smoking, drinking, drugging, porn... the list goes on. For addicts, vices can be dangerous and deadly because we don't know when to stop until it's too late. It's all about finding something else to become addicted to. I truly believe that I will always be addicted to something, so knowing that, I have chosen to become addicted to a few things since I got sober a decade ago.

The first year of recovery is intense. Find a smoker and ask them how hard it is to quit. They will gladly tell you how excruciating the experience was. Many don't quit because they don't know what to do when that craving hits. Well, let me share with you some of the things I did that helped distract me from my vices.

Six months into my recovery, I signed up for a kickboxing class. I had never boxed in my life. I heard it was an intense workout, so I found the nearest boxing gym and signed up. It was everything I thought it would be. It was tough!

At the time I was smoking about five to seven cigarettes a day. I wasn't drinking or drugging anymore. I was ready for a challenge.

I was in new town, I was newly sober, and in a new job. I didn't have friends, and my social life consisted of daily AA meetings. I went to bed at 6 pm and woke up at 2 am to be ready for the morning news. But upon reflection, that was the best thing that could have happened to me. It kept me out of trouble because by the time the weekend hit, I was too tired to stay out late. I did get the urge to go out, but just didn't have the energy.

My AA sponsor at the time told me I needed to join a club or athletic team to join to keep my mind busy during those hours of down time. Down time can be a recovering addict's worst nightmare. Down time gives us that time to think, and we addicts know that thinking is our biggest problem. I always tell people, "I don't have a drinking problem. I have a thinking problem."

I started going to kickboxing twice a week. That quickly turned into three times a week, and not too much later I was in the boxing ring five times a week. I loved it. I thrived on the action. I loved the adrenaline pumping through my veins.

The first year of sobriety was tough for me. I never experienced a pink cloud that many newly recovering addicts experience. I was in a dark space and the boxing ring gave me a space to let out that anger, sadness, frustration. It was a healthy outlet for me. About three minutes into that first training session, I couldn't breathe. I was coughing up my lungs in the corner. Everyone was looking at me. They were staring at me in disgust.

My trainer asked me, "Do you smoke?"

Ugh. I was so embarrassed. I said, "Yeah, man. I do. And I smoked my last cigarette on my way here today."

It was true that was my last cigarette. It took me getting punched in the face during an intense three-minute round against my trainer to get me to surrender to that vice. I was bragging to him before our session that I played international soccer years ago. I told my trainer I was a stellar athlete. Truth was, I was the loser in the corner hacking up a lung after three minutes. But those who know me know this: I love a good challenge. I thrive on people who don't believe in me. That fuels my fire. I love proving my doubters wrong. I quit cold turkey. Never smoked again.

But this new addiction to kickboxing began to grow into an unhealthy vice for me. It wasn't enough for me to just do the cardio kickboxing class. I wanted to spar with guys inside the ring. Keep this in mind: the fight club where I trained at in Atlanta was home to four MMA professional fighters. This was their training facility. I was surrounded by pro and amateur fighters. These were guys who had been training for years, and here I was asking to jump into the ring with them.

This played right into my defects of character: EGO. Hello, ego! My coach warned me, "Brandon. You are just starting to learn to sport. Don't jump into that ring. You are not ready. You are not ready to spar with those guys yet. Besides, you're a news anchor. You can't go into work with a busted face!"

I had played soccer in Europe and those skills came into play in kickboxing. I was training with my coach, who also happens to be a pro MMA fighter, and he was holding pads for me. He was teaching me different attacking kicks. He told me to let loose. I did exactly what he said. I whaled on him with my right kick to his upper thigh. Mind you, he was holding pads. My kick was so hard that I gave him a black and blue bruise through the pad! I had never seen my coach wince in pain.

He got up, looked at me, and said, "That is the hardest I've ever been kicked. Ever." I was proud and that only fueled my ego. Things escalated quickly.

I begged him to spar with me. He agreed under one condition: that we would spar lightly. As we began, we did spar lightly, hitting and kicking each other. But things started to escalate. I was new to the sport and I accidentally kicked him really hard. His natural reflex was to kick me back just as hard, and he did. He connected with a kick that sent me flying across the room and crashing into the side wall.

Lesson learned? Nope! He wanted to stop. I begged him to continue. We started light sparring again. Within minutes, things escalated again. He hit me hard and I kicked him back. This time the top of my foot smashed into his elbow. I broke just about every bone on the top of my foot. It swelled into the shape of a baseball.

This was the result of me not accepting my limitations. My ego getting in the way and getting me hurt. Just like drinking did. Its OK to have a drink, but it's never a good idea to binge drink. Just like in kickboxing. It was healthy for me to lightly spar and enjoy the benefits from the cardio aspect of the sport. But no, not this addict. I needed more and more until I got the shit kicked out of me.

I finally decided to hang up the boxing gloves for good and traded it in for the tennis racket. I love tennis. I think about tennis all the time. I love it because it's just me and my opponent. I am able to get into a zone. I love tennis because you can always improve. I can set new goals for myself every week. It gives me something to work toward.

Now, some people thought I was crazy when I was the only person on the tennis court in the middle of summer in Arizona when the temperature outside was 115 and the temp on the court was 124. I didn't care. I wanted to get better. I wanted to beat certain players who had beaten me. No one would hit with me in that heat, so I hit with the ball machine.

Again, my addict personality came into play. People who have played against me or those who have come to watch one of my matches will tell you that you'd think I was playing in the finals of a grand slam tournament like the US Open. I'm intense on the court. I play to win. I love the competitive fire that burns inside of me. In tennis, I really can't do myself harm. I have only experienced healthy benefits from it.

When I became obsessed with kickboxing, my sponsor saw I was still struggling with addiction and said to me, "Brandon, we really need you to find a healthy habit to keep your mind busy when you're not at the gym or at work. We have got to keep you busy every minute of every day. You cannot afford to have down time like normal folks."

I remember how broke I was at the time. I didn't have any money saved up. I couldn't afford to decorate my home. So I walked into a nearby art gallery and stared at artwork for hours. I asked the worker at the gallery how much one of the paintings was and about flatlined when she said, "That piece is listed at $115,000."

Jesus! That was ludicrous. I said to myself, "Are you kidding me? Hell, I can go home an paint that!" Welcome back Mr. Ego!

I walked out of that art gallery and Googled the nearest art store. I walked in, grabbed a couple canvases on sale, and bought some acrylic paints. I walked home and laid everything out. I opened the tubes of paint and I began to recreate what I had seen in the gallery. I quickly realized that it wasn't as easy as it looked. Shocker. But I really enjoyed it. I looked at the clock and realized that five hours had just passed. It felt like I had been painting for 30 minutes. Not five hours!

This was exactly the kind of hobby I needed. Something I enjoyed doing and help pass the down time. I had no idea where that curiosity would eventually lead me. Over the course of my time in Atlanta, I realized that my art would disappear off my walls. My friends were taking them. They asked me, "B, where did you buy this art?" I told them I created it all. They were shocked because I never spoke about art. Ever.

When people find out I paint, they ask "Brandon, when did you learn to paint?"

My answer: "I just learned. I picked up some paint and canvases. That's it!"

One day a friend came over and wandered down into my basement. He screamed, "Brandon! Come down here now!" I walked downstairs and said, "What are you doing down here? No one is supposed to be down here."

My friend looked at me with his jaw dropped. "Brandon, did you paint all of these?"

"Yes, I did. I have to take them all to the dumpster and throw them out. They're all mistakes and mess ups."

He looked at me and said, "Like hell you will throw these out. I will take them all. Don't you dare throw them out."

My friend had a plan. He called one of his friends who happened to own an art gallery. My friend knew that I would never agree to let anyone else see the artwork. I was insecure about it. I didn't think it was good enough. I would finish a piece and only recognize the mistakes. That's exactly how I viewed my life. I wasn't able to recognize the good in me, only the mistakes I had made. The scars of my vices.

My friend's plan involved getting access to my paintings while I was at work. He told me he needed to stay at my house for the day while his home was being repaired. I didn't think twice about it. While I was at work, he invited his friend, the gallery owner, to my house. They went into the basement and viewed all of my artwork that was days from being in a landfill.

According to my friend, the gallery owner flipped out. He told my friend NOT to allow me to throw it away. Instead, he begged me to donate it to charity since I was going to dump it anyway. I agreed. He took the art and to my surprise, over the next six months, every one of those pieces sold at auction. I couldn't understand how that was possible. Why would anyone want that art with all those mistakes? Because, just like me, people in my life today love and accept me for my scars. It's a lesson that's taken me years to understand.

Art infuses me with light and life. I can spend eight to ten hours inside my art studio. The outside world doesn't matter to me in those moments. I thrive during that once dreaded down time. My mind goes into a creative space. Music is blaring. I'm in the zone. Sometimes I start a piece, and by the time I'm done, it has turned into something totally different.

Art has taught me to not be so black and white about everything. If something doesn't work out the way I had envisioned, that's OK. Perhaps it will lead me to something even better and more beautiful. Another life lesson: don't throw something away or dismiss it for its flaws. Instead, find the beauty in it.

My therapist taught me this when she asked me this pointed question: "Brandon, when will you begin to see yourself the way the rest of us see you?"

I asked her, "What do you see when you look at me and my life?"

"I see someone who is loving, compassionate, creative, thoughtful, encouraging, positive... why are you laughing, Brandon?"

"Sorry, I'm laughing because I'm uncomfortable hearing you say those things about me."

"Why?" she asked.

All I could say was, "I don't know. I guess I just don't see myself that way."

My artwork went from being an experiment to keep my mind busy during that dreaded down time to a hobby to a second business. I have sold paintings to people all over the globe. I have been blessed to have my work featured in major hotel lobbies. I still laugh about the time when a gallery called me to tell me, "Justin Bieber is here with his designer and they love your artwork. You just sold a piece to the Biebs!"

When people tell me, "I wish I could paint. I wish could draw. I can't even draw a good stick figure," I tell them my story. I tell them art is more than a paint brush and acrylics. Art is all around us. You have a phone. Take pictures of cool things you see while walking down the street. Print that picture and paint on top of it. Give it texture. Who cares if you mess up. I never got into art to make money. Far from it. Art literally saved me from a relapse. It occupied my mind for eight hours a day during that first year of recovery.

We are all artists. Tap into that creativity even if you never show a single person what you've created. Just create. Use bright colors. Use dark colors. Do things that scare you. Do things that force you to make mistakes, so that you eventually shrug a shoulder to an error. Soon enough you will begin to embrace mistakes as beautiful texture in your life.

Instead of trying to reprogram my addictive personality, I took a vice and turned it into something healthy. I can't stop playing tennis. I can't stop thinking about my next art project. That's all healthy stuff. At least I'm no longer saying, "I can't stop getting high. I can't stop thinking about my next fix."

9

Red Flag Warning in Effect

It was Memorial Day Weekend, 2012. I had more than two years sober at the time. I told you about my sponsor's rule in year one: no dating. Well, I successfully passed that test. I was open to dating but I certainly wasn't on the hunt for a boyfriend. I spent that holiday in Pensacola, Florida, at a huge gay party weekend on the beach. I was there with a bunch of my friends. It was a beautiful place to vacation. The sand was silky-white smooth. The water was turquoise and crystal clear. It was majestic. We were hanging out by the pool which overlooked the ocean. A DJ spun some fun dance beats in the background. Guys were dancing everywhere. The sun was shining. The temperature was 75. It was a slice of heaven.

That's when I laid eyes on him. This guy with a chiseled body and a masculine aura. He had confidence. Swagger. We made eye contact but he kept walking. I wasn't about to let him get away. I followed him and said, "Hey, man! What's your name?"

"My name is Jackson," he replied in a thick country accent. I am one of those people who is sucker for an accent. British. Australian. But most of all a southern accent is like game, set, match.

We chatted for a couple minutes and I offered, "Can I give you my number?"

He didn't seem impressed. It was as if he felt obliged to accept it. We walked to the bar and I scribbled my name and number onto a napkin and I handed it to him. He told me he lived in North Georgia, about an hour outside of Atlanta. He went his way. I went my way. That was it. I never heard from him. I was anxiously awaiting a text message all weekend. But the weekend turned into a week turned into a month. Nothing. I was bummed because there was something about this guy that I was drawn to.

Labor Day weekend rolled around and I went to a friend's birthday party. He rented the entire upstairs of a restaurant. When I drank and drugged, I used to be the life of the party. I would talk to anyone about anything.

Sober, however, I am much more of an introvert. I can talk openly for hours about intimate subjects with people I know. But I don't enjoy small talk with people I don't know. Sometimes, people assume I'm not a nice guy. Time and time again my friends will tell other guys, "Brandon is a really warm and nice guy, you just have to get to know him."

My friends would say this in my defense when other guys approached them asking why I rarely talked to people I didn't know. Part of it was that I had just two years of sobriety at the time and I was still learning how to be social in an environment where people were drinking and I was not. I challenge you to go to a party and not have one drink and then you'll realize what it's like for a sober person to talk with people who are buzzed or wasted. It's not very fun.

So, I'm at this birthday party. People are dancing, having a great time. I went to the bathroom but the door was locked, so I waited outside. Then the door swung open and my jaw dropped. It was Jackson. The guy I met briefly in Pensacola who had taken my breath away.

He recognized me and gave me a smirk. I panicked and just said, "Hey, man," and went into the bathroom. Smooth B, really smooth.

I contemplated if I should find him at the party and talk with him. I left the bathroom and saw him standing across the room. We made eye contact. I did something brave for me: I walked up to him and started the conversation. I asked him why he hadn't called me.

He said, "I thought you were way too pretty for me."

I was flattered. He had this smooth Southern charm. A charm that would win over a jury in a criminal case. I was drawn to him, but I still couldn't figure out why. This was the first time in recovery that I had those butterflies in my stomach for someone. It was a real infatuation. A crush.

This was the first time I had considered being in a relationship since becoming sober. No more anonymous sex. No more having sex while being high. No more navigating a relationship based on just sex and drugs. This is was going to be my first grown-up relationship, and like new relationships other people have in their youth, I was naive and totally unprepared. I had hormones dictating my actions and emotions clouding my judgment.

We decided to go on that first date. He offered to take me hiking the next day up in North Georgia. I didn't hesitate. I canceled my brunch plans with friends and told them, "Sorry, y'all. I'm going on a date with that hot guy I told you about!"

We met at a hiking trail about 45 minutes outside the city. He rolled up in a lifted Ford F-150 truck. Damn. This guy seemed to know my biggest weaknesses: Southern accent, charm, and a lifted off-road truck. The hike was lovely. I got to see parts of the state that I had never experienced. He led the way and we talked about everything.

I even told him about my two-plus years in recovery and what my life used to be like and what my life is like today. He seemed cool about it. It didn't seem to scare him off. We finished the hike and chatted in the parking lot. I didn't want the date to end, but I also didn't know what to say to extend it.

Apparently he felt the same way. He was brave enough to

ask me, "Do you want to come see my ranch? It's only about 20 minutes from here."

I tried hard to contain my excitement and said, "Most definitely. I'm up for it."

We hopped into his truck and headed down a dirt road. He asked, "You mind if we make a pit stop real quick?"

We pulled up in front of this beat-down shack that had a glowing neon sign out front that read Cold Beers. Mind you, we had just gone a two-hour hike and during this long two hours we talked about a lot of stuff, including my battle with addiction. He jumped out of the truck and said, "I'll be right back."

I had butterflies, but this time it was a nervous butterfly. He walked out of the liquor store five minutes later carrying a 24-case of Natural Ice beer. I wanted to gag.

My first thought was, *Seriously? Natty Ice? Who drinks that shit? He clearly has bad taste in beer.* He hopped in the truck and off we went to his ranch. We drove down another long dirt road and all of a sudden the overgrown trees broke open at the very end, revealing a gorgeous hand-built ranch house overlooking a tranquil private lake. It reminded me of a scene from the romantic classic, *The Notebook.*

He drove me around the property, which was huge. His entire family lived on this massive property. I don't even know how many acres it was. Each family member had their own ranch house built on the land. It was so big you couldn't even see the other houses.

We walked into his ranch and chatted for a bit on his couch.

One thing led to another to another, and the next thing you know we were having passionate sex. Guys in sobriety always told me, "Brandon, sober sex is the best sex. Promise. One day you'll experience it."

I was incredulous. There was no way sober sex can be better than drug sex. For the first time, I finally understood what those guys were trying to tell me. Not only was the sex good, but the connection was intense. Sober, you feel every sense. Every touch. Every deep stare into your partner's eyes.

After sex, he invited me to take a hot shower with him. In my opinion, there is nothing more intimate than being totally naked with someone in the shower after sex. I felt totally comfortable naked with another man for the first time in my life. I wasn't scared. I wasn't insecure. I felt incredible. I was falling for this guy.

Then, all of the sudden, Jackson said, "Stay here. I will be right back."

He hopped out of the shower, naked and soaking wet. I heard the refrigerator door slam and footsteps running back to the shower. He hopped in holding two beers. He cracked one open, and just like my college drinking days, shotgunned the beer and guzzled it down in three seconds. He crushed the can with his fist, let out a huge burp, and started laughing.

I was frozen. I wasn't sure what to do. Do I run out of that house? Do I stay and pretend I'm ok? He then went in for a kiss.

I could taste the beer in his mouth. I thought to myself, *Goddamn, this is so hot*, knowing full well that I was in danger. You know the movie *Ghost* when Whoopie says to Demi, "Molly, you in danger, girl!" That should have been the biggest red flag.

Just hours before the hot steamy shower, we were on a hiking trail and I was pouring my heart out, telling this guy about my struggles with addiction in the past, and he swings by a liquor store, shotguns two beers in front of me, and then kisses me. Seriously? Why couldn't I see the red flags? Sadly, things were about to get worse. I was acting like stupid prepubescent teen. All hormones, no sense.

We dated for the next few months and the red flags were visible to everyone except me. I didn't see them because I didn't want to see them. I rationalized that everything was great. I felt great. I was not drinking, and everything was fine. He was an adult and he could make his own choices and that it would not have any effect on me or my sobriety.

Jackson rarely came down to the city to hang out with me and my friends. He wanted to be alone, or he only wanted to hang out with his friends in North Georgia. He got drunk all the time and I became his personal driver to and from the bars. Oh, how fun. But he would win me over with his charm when he sensed that I was growing tired of his antics.

He would make me dinner. Let me tell you, Jackson knew how to cook a traditional Southern meal with all the fixings. As he prepared dinner one Sunday night, I was at the counter texting Hannah. After our first encounter when I moved to Atlanta, we had become extremely close; she was and is my sister. She is part of my chosen family. She has almost 20 years sober and has always guided me through life's issues as they happen.

I was texting with her—I don't even know what we were talking about—and Jackson noticed what I was doing. The look on his face was not one of delight. No. Jackson was pissed.

"Who you talkin' to?" he asked.

"Hannah. She just texted and we're chatting."

"What are you guys talking about?" he asked.

"Stuff. Nothing major."

"Then tell me what you're talking about," Jackson insisted.

"Don't worry about it. We're not talking about you. She's someone I can talk to about anything. She gets me. She's sober. She just gets me and we can talk about anything. She's my person."

Something shifted. Something dangerous was triggered in Jackson, and this was just the tip of the iceberg.

"Oh, hell no. I am your person. Not Hannah. If you got something to talk about, then you talk about it with me. Not her!"

Oh, fuck. Was he kidding? Nope. He wasn't kidding. His face was bright red and he was holding a large kitchen knife. What I didn't realize was that Jackson had been isolating me. He was a master at charm and manipulation. He didn't want me talking to my best friend. He didn't want me to have any friend that in any way challenged his dominion over me. That was not a good sign. Jackson was essentially training me. I was to go to him when I had any problems because he wanted me to depend only on him.

It didn't make sense to me at the time why he would have such a problem with Hannah. If anything, you'd think my boyfriend would want to give her a hug and say, "Thank you for saving him so I can enjoy him and his company." Nope. That was not what Jackson had in mind. I was his possession and he was not sharing.

The more time I spent with Jackson, though, I became more aware of this Jekyll & Hyde persona. Jackson had a beautiful pit bull named Booker. Booker was a sweet dog. Always loving. Always nearby. Jackson turned around one day and grabbed Booker by the collar and said to him, "I am going to take you out into the woods and tie you up to a tree and leave you there for days until you're starving and then you'll find out who's boss."

Booker didn't do anything to be treated that way. But, I realized that I was in the same boat as Booker. I was just another dog for him to dominate and possess. I was in trouble, yet still I stayed.

One night I was in the bathroom and the door was propped open. I was brushing my teeth before crashing to bed and I glanced in the bathroom mirror and noticed a chilling figure in that far background staring at me. It was Jackson. Have you ever seen the movie *Sleeping with the Enemy?* In it Julia Roberts played the role of an abused wife. She was trapped, and in the end she almost lost her life, because her crazed husband would not let her go. That's the feeling I got at that moment. Not a warm fuzzy mesmerizing stare. This was a cold-hearted mean stare as if he were fantasizing about ways to kill me. Still, I stayed because I learned very early on in life that abuse and love can coexist. I can thank my mom for that life lesson.

About a week later, Jackson and I got into an argument. He told me, in front of his entire family, that AA was a cult. That recovery was stupid. In my mind my boyfriend should have been my biggest supporter in recovery. Why was he bashing me and my sobriety and doing it in front of his family?

I was ashamed. I was embarrassed. I was also pissed off. I broke up with him that night and swore I would never go back.

Addicts are good at lying and making empty promises. The ones they make the biggest promises to, and fail to deliver to, are themselves. Even though I was no longer an active addict, I was still trying to figure out this life thing—with a clear mind, which I did not have much practice doing. I did what I knew best; I was about to make a promise I had no intention of keeping.

Two weeks later, I was driving down that long dirt road to Jackson's ranch. I walked into the house and the smell of food overtook my senses. It also wiped away the anger I had. Jackson's charm won me over.

But not for long. In fact, the warmth lasted about 20 minutes. At first it was great. I apologized for leaving him. He never apologized. He only hugged me and said, "Don't ever leave me again."The alarms rang louder than ever. *Get out, B. Run and never look back.* I stayed.

He turned around to finish cooking and I laid down on his bed. The next thing I knew, Jackson jumped on me, pinning me down. He's 6'3". I'm 5'11". He weighed about 200 pounds. I weighed about 170. It wasn't hard for him to hold me down. He then raised his right arm as if he was an MMA fighter about to deal a vicious blow. There was this evil look in his eyes. A cruel hard look that he meant business. "Don't you ever fucking leave me again like that or I will fucking beat you."

I truly thought he was going to kill me. He got off me and walked back into the kitchen, laughing hysterically. I was terrified. Mortified. That's when I felt my higher power, my guardian angel, stirring in my breast. Something came over me and lifted me off that bed. I grabbed my phone and keys and I ran for the front door. I buzzed by Jackson in the kitchen. He was caught off guard, which gave me a couple of seconds to escape. I ran to my truck. Hopped in. Started the engine.

I threw my truck into reverse and there he was. Jackson, staring directly at me. I threw my truck into drive and sped off. I saw him run back inside and I was sure he was going to chase me. He did know where I lived, after all. I sped down the freeway going 90 miles an hour.

I was sobbing. Tears streamed down my face. I called my

sponsor, CeCe. She always knew exactly what to say and how to help me when I needed it the most. She told me I needed to call a locksmith immediately to change all the locks at my house. Within 90 minutes my locks were changed.

Here's one of the important messages I learned through all of this: My best friend Hannah was there for me the entire time. This was not my first breakup with Jackson, but it was my last. Jackson and I had entered a vicious cycle of breaking up and getting back together. Hannah had to watch me cry over and over again. She never once told me to leave him. In fact, she did the opposite. I would complain to her how bad of a guy Jackson was, but in the same breath would tell her, "But I love him and I know he loves me, too." Denial is a tough river to navigate.

Hannah looked me in the eyes and told me, "Brandon, you're not done yet. You need to go back to him. The only way this will ever end is when you've finally hit rock bottom with him. You're not there yet. Go back." She knew me so well.

She did ask me to promise her one thing. "B, you have to go to an AA meeting once a day. That's it. Go back with Jackson, but as your best friend make me a promise that you will continue to hit AA meetings through this."

That was easy. My best friend just gave me the ok to go back with Jackson; hitting an AA meeting daily was no big task at all. I enjoyed sobriety meetings. Two weeks later, Jackson raised his fist to me. Hannah knew that if I stayed connected to AA and the people in recovery, it would only be a matter of time for ME to realize that Jackson was no good for me.

Hannah knew that if she said, "Brandon you have to break up with Jackson…." it would have only driven me back to him sooner and would have likely damaged our friendship because people often choose an abusive husband or partner over their friends. Hannah knew that, which is why she never tried to convince me to leave him. Hannah encouraged me to keep the positive things in my life, meetings and friends, and not to isolate.

I guess that is what threatened Jackson about Hannah. She knew me and how I processed information. She was smart, she could see through his facade, and he knew if anyone could talk me out of my relationship with him, it was Hannah. Even though she did not do it directly, she sensed me isolating, and threw me a life raft to keep for when I needed it.

Sure enough, I left Jackson that last time and I never went back. I did run into him on the streets a few years later and my heart never sank, never skipped a beat. It was nothing. I was done. He was another ugly addiction that I had rid myself of. His negative energy was palpable. I couldn't believe that I wanted to be with him. The man I am today isn't even attracted to that negative energy. But for my entire life up until that time, I always knew I had a bad picker. I gravitated toward guys who were no good. My therapist bluntly told me one day, "Jackson is your mother." Chilling.

How to deal with Toxic Family

Here's the litmus test for every relationship, friendship or intimate, that I have in my life. Yes, this includes family members. You're either pushing me closer to my spiritual center, or you're pulling me away from it. If you bring me close to that inner peace and spirituality, then you stay in my life. If you tear me away from that inner peace, then I am letting you go.

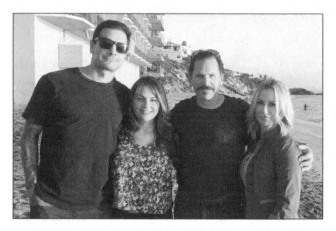

From Left: Me, my sister Stephanie, my dad, my sister Catherine

That litmus test has been my saving grace. I had to use that litmus test for my sister Catherine. I love her. She's my sister. She's blood. But she's a terribly abusive person. She was the most verbally abusive person in my life growing up. She would berate me in front of people. She made life miserable for me. Living with her in the house was like walking on eggshells.

When I was 33, I moved to Phoenix for a new job. Catherine wanted to come visit me. I didn't really want her to, but I thought to myself, *You know, Brandon, give her another chance.* So I did. Catherine came to visit, and sure enough, 24 hours into her stay we had our first and last argument.

Catherine has been cut off by my mother and my sister. The only person who still communicates with her is my dad. Parents will do anything to help their child. It's human instinct for a parent to sacrifice themselves for their child, even if that child is abusive to them. But I'm her brother. I don't have those instincts to force myself into that abusive relationship.

We were at dinner and my sister brought up our mother. Catherine was bad-mouthing her for hours. Now, dealing with my mom is no walk in the park. She too has bipolar characteristics. But I had enough. I told Catherine, "Your relationship with mom is your relationship with mom. My relationship with mom is my relationship with mom. Not yours. Don't talk bad about mom to me. You keep that to yourself and your therapist. You're trying to get me to take sides and I am not going to do that."

Well, that's all Catherine needed to hear. We drove home from the restaurant and she packed up her stuff and she drove six hours home to California in the dead of the night. Five years have passed since her visit. The few communications I have received have been in the form of venom-filled, alcohol-inspired text messages.

Hateful and hurtful. I never replied. It has only solidified that I am healthier with her on the outside of my life.

But the fact is, Catherine is mentally ill. I don't mean that in a disparaging way. She is truly sick. I don't want to ever be mean or hurtful to someone who is suffering, but that also doesn't mean I have to stick around to be abused either. I can love from far away. I have learned through the help of my incredible therapist that I can create healthy boundaries and not apologize or feel guilty for doing so.

Catherine recently asked to talk on the phone. I told her, "I love you. I just don't know how I can move forward yet."

I mentioned to my dad that I received a message from Catherine. He informed me that she had attempted suicide and was in the hospital. I told my dad, "Dad, I love you. I know you are trying everything you can do help Catherine. I don't blame you or disparage you from your instincts as a father. This is going to sound cold, but it's the truth. If she really wanted to kill herself, she would have done it. This is a cry for help, but will she get the help she needs this time? Or is she going to play victim again, and blame all of us for her problems?"

I go back to my litmus test: Is Catherine pushing me toward my spiritual center? Fuck no. Is she pulling me away from it? Fuck yes. So for me the decision is difficult, yet simple. Until Catherine gets the help she needs OR admits to me that she has a problem with alcohol or mental illness, then there is nothing I can do to save her. All I can do is choose to protect me. She abused me enough as a kid and yes, even as an adult until I finally got the courage to cut her off. I am choosing my own spiritual center over my sister and I have no guilt about it.

FIND ROMEO

I'm not a psychologist, but I have had multiple therapists tell me that my mother is bipolar and a narcissist. Like my sister, she is sick. While I have empathy, that does not mean I have not built up huge boundaries to protect myself. She can never admit she is wrong and does not really have compassion for other people, especially her children. I talked to my therapist about my family reading this book and what impact it might have on my life and my relationship with them.

I am tired of living the life of my youth. Afraid. Abused. Controlled.

What is the worst my parents can do to me? Write me out of the will? I am not some cheap politician who can be paid for and controlled. No more. Not today.

I grew up listening to the language of guilt.

"Look at everything we provided. The best home. The best neighborhood. The best schools and athletic programs. You owe us."

While I am appreciative for what my parents provided me,

it does not balance the scales. I was emotionally and at times physically abused by my mother. I often would walk around scared about the next time she would scream at me or hit me. My mom was a black belt in Karate. I will never forget one night she was on the phone with a client at the kitchen table. Apparently, I was being a typical 7 year old being loud in the family room. She flipped. She lost it. Before I even had a chance to run, my mom took a knife that was sitting on the table and hurled it toward me like a Japanese throwing star. It was coming at me in slow motion. But I was frozen. Scared. Terrified. That knife slashed the wooden wall behind my head. It was that type of abuse, control, manipulation that I am finally free from.

In AA it is important that you make amends in your life and try to heal relationships. In theory, it is a noble undertaking. But in the reality of my life, it was torture.

My first AA sponsor suggested that I call my parents on a regular basis.

"My parents never call me about my recovery. Why should I call them?"

My sponsor would not accept this answer, so he gave me an assignment.

"You must call your parents every week."

There is this idea that you should make amends so that when they pass away, there is no unfinished business and guilt. I did as instructed and called them daily.

"Hey, Mom, how are you?" I began my conversations. She then launched into some tirade about her work and her life. She never asked how I was doing. She never asked about my recovery. Not a word about any new relationship in my life. It was all about her.

I would end each conversation with, "I love you."

Her response was often, "Ok." And then she hung up.

This went on for years. Finally I connected with a fantastic therapist and I told her about my weekly call and how it was making me feel terrible. She was shocked and horrified. I was this thirsty kid looking for water, and I was going to the same well, week after week, hoping to satiate myself. I would lower the bucket into the well and only return with dry sand.

"How many more times are you going to go to that dry well?" my therapist asked me. "There will never be any water in there for you."

She was right and gave me permission to stop calling my mother. I was torturing myself with the belief that after so many years, my parents would change. I have no regrets.

To illustrate how toxic my mother was in my life, I want share with you the story of Romeo. My mother was a successful real estate agent and decided one day to run for city council in Orange County. She did it solely because she had a vendetta against some of the other candidates.

I was living in Atlanta at the time, having left Los Angeles.

Remember, I worked as a reporter in LA for a few years, so people in the business knew who I was. One day I received a call from my ex who told me that my mother was on the local news.

"Excuse me?" I replied.

"You have got to see this. I am going to send you the link now," he informed me.

The lead was, city council candidate in Orange County puts up a $50,000 reward to find her lost chihuahua, which she claims was stolen by her city council opponent.

I was mortified. She was on two news channels where I had worked, telling her story. She called in the FBI to investigate. She had totally lost all touch with reality. The news stations were having a field day with it. They thought she was crazy, and she had become a laughingstock.

I returned to my parent's home soon after this. I walked into the kitchen and two things struck me. The first was a large TV monitor with images from 16 different video cameras around the house. The second was a herd of about 10 chihuahuas running and barking in the living room.

There was my mother sitting in a chair with about five of them in her lap saying over and over, "Oh I love you, I love you," as they licked her face.

"You just told those dogs you love them more times in 30 seconds than you ever told me in my entire life," were the words that came out of my mouth.

She just glared at me.

"What the hell is going on? You went to my old station for an interview? You are a joke to them and an embarrassment to me. People think you are nuts."

She didn't care. My sister got a call from the FBI because they were worried my mom might send a "package" to her opponent. Things had gotten way out of hand. And I was done being part of that madness.

When I returned to Atlanta, I changed my last name to Lee, which was my middle name. I no longer wanted to be associated with her. She sent me care packages with bumper stickers she had made up that said, "Where's Romeo?" Yes, the name of the missing dog was Romeo.

She asked a few of my childhood friends to go around to shelters to look for Romeo. One of them called me and said, "B, I would love to help out, if that is what you want me to do. But seriously, this is California. Do you know how many chihuahuas there are here?"

I told them to call her back and tell her they had looked but had no luck.

People ask me why I changed my name and I tell them that Lee is an easier name to say and remember. The truth is I did not want anyone to associate me with her anymore.

I was also angry at my father, and I did confront him. He knew about the abuse from my mom and my sister and did nothing. I would call him at work when I was a child and beg him to help me because my sister was hurting me. He ignored it. He was too busy working to provide me the best of everything.

Isn't it a parent's job to protect their children? It is not about sending them to the best schools and buying them fancy clothes; it is about caring for their well-being, and my father had failed. I told him how I felt, and he was silent.

Then he said, "Give me a week to digest it and then we'll talk."

I do believe he was sorry, but he lacked the will to do anything about it, then or now. He knew that my mother had been verbally and physically abusive to me and yet he continued to stick by her. I don't care if they get divorced. I cannot accept that he stayed with her so I would have an intact family when he knew how cruel she is.

Over the years I have received calls from my father, crying. "I think she is going to kill me, Brandon."

Leave. For God's sake, leave her.

"You are a grown man in your sixties. You still have a life. Leave her. Find someone else who will make you happy and who you can travel with. Find your true soulmate."

I finally refused to listen to it and said, "Stop crying about it and just get the hell out. I can't give you any other advice."

Family is not easy. We fight. We bicker. We get on each other's nerves. I envy my friends who have incredibly close families. I want that for me one day. The reality is that I have to rid myself of my birth family's toxicity in order to create my own family. There is no way I can have toxic family members in my life and bring my future husband around that. I would NEVER subject my future husband to that. Ever. If I did, then I would be the abuser.

PITFALLS OF RELATIONSHIPS DURING RECOVERY

Making friends when you're drinking and drugging is easy. You walk into a bar. You have a few drinks. You feel buzzed. Liquid courage sets in and you start introducing yourself to total strangers. These strangers soon become "friends" you meet up with for a good time. I always thought of myself as the life of the party. Heck, what addict doesn't?

I considered myself to be an extrovert. I would go up to anyone and strike up a conversation at a club or bar. The friends I made during my active addiction I thought were some of the best friends anyone could hope for. It was guaranteed to be a fun time. Every Friday night at 11 pm we would meet up in West Hollywood and we would hit all the bars. The first bar we always met up at was a bar called Eleven in the heart of WeHo.

I wasn't a drinker, so I would usually do a dose of GHB in my truck. I'd wait ten minutes to feel the buzz, then I would walk into the bar. We would travel the world together in large groups. We'd travel to exotic places. We travelled on cruise ships dubbed Drug Tugs. Imagine four thousand gay men crammed onto a cruise ship in the middle of the ocean. What could possibly happen?

It was all fun until it wasn't. Near-death experiences are real buzz kills.

As I became sober, I realized how hollow those friendships really were. Don't get me wrong, I had a fun time partying with the guys in Hollywood, but the reality is chilling: The moment I got sober, I lost 95% of my "friends." Newly sober, I wasn't meeting up with the crew on Friday nights to rage. These friends will call you once, maybe twice to meet up. If you don't meet up with them, suddenly the phone stops ringing and the invites stop coming.

The WeHo guys I hung out with had this attitude: "What have you done for me lately?" If you don't have drugs to share or aren't willing to drink into a blackout, these guys didn't have a need for you. Getting sober is lonely at the beginning. Addicts often mourn the loss of our old life and our old friends. Take away the booze and drugs and the truth is, we didn't have much in common. I didn't know much about these guys anyway. I knew the music they liked and the drugs they took. I didn't know anything about their lives beyond that.

The hard truth is, if you want to become sober and stay sober, you have to choose new playgrounds and new playmates. I became morose and thought I'd never laugh or have fun again. I thought people would refuse to hang out with me because I was sober.

How fun can a sober guy be anyway? I was about to find out.

In AA, they encourage you to fellowship with other addicts. After meetings, most of the guys would go out for food or coffee. It was a way for addicts to get to know other addicts. From my experience at meetings, I watched a lot of guys fellowship. In fact, for many of the guys in the rooms of AA, those meetings became their total existence. They only hung out with people in the rooms. The outside world was scary to them. They felt safe in AA. That's great for many of these guys because to them, just making it through the day without taking a drink is a huge success.

I wanted more. As often as my sponsors encouraged me to fellowship, I never did. I had maybe two real friends in recovery who I'd fellowship with and hang out with. Some guys wrote me off saying, "Oh, Brandon is too cool to hang with us." As I've said before, the rooms of AA can sometimes be a super judgmental place. Gay guys in general can be catty. Hell, I am guilty of it, too!

I wanted to connect with people outside the confines of the AA rooms. I didn't get sober to just hang out with sober people. I got sober to enjoy life with normies. Consider that there is a great number of people who are struggling with drugs or booze and will never find the rooms of AA. So, I believe my higher calling is to simply be an example to others that no matter how far down the scale they have fallen, they too can have healthy relationships, successful careers, and a fulfilling life.

It didn't take long for me to rid myself of toxic friendships.

In fact, it happened quite naturally. My party friends stopped calling because I stopped showing up to party on Friday nights. When I walked into AA, my life immediately changed for the good. Within a few weeks I met my first normie friend who would end up being one of my best friends to this day. His name is Jason.

I met Jason when I was 90 days sober, living in Atlanta. At first I was very quiet and shy. I would stand in the corner of the room at a house party not sure what to do. When I hit 8 months clean, I remember going with a group of friends to a popular bar. I thought I could handle it. But, I clearly wasn't ready. I didn't even notice my body having an adverse reaction.

Jason came up to me and asked, "Brandon, are you OK?"

"Yea, why you ask?" I replied.

"You are gripping this iron fence and your knuckles are white!"

My inner soul was recoiling like a hot flame from the old party scene. At the time, I didn't want to look weak, so I said I was fine. Jason was a true friend who cared about me. He looked at me and said, "Brandon, we're leaving. This is not safe for you. Let's go."

That's a real friend. He didn't care that he wouldn't be partying on a Friday night. He cared more about my safety than himself!

It's quite humorous to see the reaction of my current friends' faces when I tell them a war story from my drinking days. They sit there in disbelief. They cannot imagine me being so wild and out of control. Remember, the friends in my life today have only ever known me sober, so they get to experience a much better version of me than when I chose drugs and alcohol above everything else.

"Brandon, you are the most in-control person I have ever met. There's no way you did that," they say.

That, to me, is the best compliment I could receive. It's taken so much work to change from the man I used to be. I don't take all the credit, though. My higher power has given me the courage and the strength to face my demons and fight back. Without the spirituality aspect of recovery, I would have nothing.

As an addict, we are a selfish lot. I care only about what you can do for me, and if you can't get me what I need, then you are of no use to me. It's brutal. It's harsh. It's the reality of being friends with an addict. You can only imagine the crowd I ran with.

Now that I am sober and have changed my outlook on life, I have naturally attracted positive people into my life. Like a magnet, I attracted quality people because I was finally behaving like a quality person. Like attracts like. My inner circle is filled with people who are caring, compassionate, thoughtful, successful, and loving.

When we're at our worst drinking and drugging, we ruin a lot of relationships. Our families get tired of us draining their bank accounts. They get tired of us showing up hungover at family dinners. When I work with a new addict in recovery, they often want to immediately say "I'm sorry" to everyone. I have to remind them that making amends is the 9th step out of 12. When you walk into the AA rooms, you are on step 1. Mending relationships takes time, and it takes a lot more than "I'm sorry."

I tell everyone we fix broken relationships by focusing on us first. Until we fix our own issues, we can't expect others to forgive us. And by cleaning up our side of the street first, we are able to show through action that we are a changed person. When our families, friends, and life partners see us working hard on removing our defects of character that hurt so many people, that's when forgiveness takes place. Actions, not words, and patience are the key ingredients to mending relationships.

Most of the amends I have made in recovery came at a time when I had nine months sober. So I had some time under my belt. I was going to meetings every day. I was doing step work with my sponsor. I was taking action. So when I made my amends, I was able to tell my family, my friends, and former coworkers that I had been working to change my behavior. I apologized to everyone on my amends list (I believe I had about 50 people on that list). I didn't just apologize, though. A true amends is asking each person I have wronged what I can do to make it right. Almost every person said the same thing: "Brandon, continue to stay sober and become the man we all know you can be. That's all I want."

It's amazing how no one asked me to repay the debts I owed. No one asked me to do anything crazy. I would have done it, by the way. I would have done just about anything to save those relationships. Instead, they just wanted me to live the life of a man with purpose, dignity, and hope. Who could ask anything more?

Sobriety has taught me so many life lessons. It's forced me to recognize what my character defects are and to be aware of them creeping into my life. One of my defects is my ability to be a chameleon. If I'm around a bunch of negative people who want to jump off a cliff to their death, I would get dark thoughts, too. Sobriety taught me how to turn that defect into a strength. If I surround myself with happy and positive people, then my life's choices are happy and positive.

It's that simple. Too bad it took me an abusive relationship and years of recovery to finally see the light.

10

Living The Sober Life

When I chose to leave my job as the main anchor for the number one station in Arizona, people asked me, "Why? What are you going to do next? What are you going to do in between jobs?"

I sat down with a reporter from the *Arizona Republic*, a newspaper similar to the *New York Times* as far as respect for quality reporting. I know how the media works. We take the most salacious part of the story and run with it.

I was honest in answering. Most anchors, reporters, and news stations lie through their teeth when someone leaves, quits, or is fired. But that's not the man I am today. I lived most of my life trying to deceive people. Trying to tell them what I thought they wanted to hear. Telling people only things that make me look good. Shit, scroll through Instagram and watch how most people try to make their lives seem absolutely perfect. It's not reality. It's not authentic. It's fakery, but people consume it like it's their last supper.

Why did I decide to leave Phoenix? It's one of the biggest news markets in the country, number 12 out of 200+ markets. Why would I give up that seat when I had so much success? These are really good questions. I've had the most success career-wise in Arizona than anywhere else I've ever worked: Boston, Atlanta, Hartford, even Los Angeles. The better question is, how could I have so much success in a state where I struggled to live personally? I've always felt like a fish out of water. I always felt out of place in Arizona, but the viewers still connected with me. Why was that?

I finally found the answer through the thousands of comments I received when I announced that I was leaving my job. People wrote me messages thanking me for sharing about my struggles with depression, addiction, and sex abuse. People appreciated me opening up about my struggles because it made them feel like they were not alone. It made them feel like they're not crazy. It almost validated for them that even people like me—a successful news anchor—struggle at times in life. So many news anchors try to portray this perfect life on social media. Partly because their bosses tell them too. Partly out of fear that if they share something "ugly," they will get in trouble.

As a society, we really have to stop looking at people who've suffered traumatic experiences in their life as if they are damaged goods. Instead, we have to look at these people as survivors, and we have to look at people who've gone through traumatic stuff as someone who is special. We have to view their disclosure of what has happened to them as the brave and courageous act it is, and embrace them in their healing and recovery.

People who have experienced trauma or made bad life choices in the past can shed new light on the topic or give us a vantage point to see an issue from a different perspective. Often, these people have much they can teach us. These are heroes who can save others from making these same mistakes and help protect them by shedding light into the darkness.

The more that we hide our scars and hide our bruises from society, the more we feed the idea that they are Pariahs of society. That we should brand them with a scarlet letter and avoid or push them out of proper society. The result is that these victims are revictimized, ostracized, and will seek any and all means to quell their pain.

As more of us who have suffered these traumatic experiences come forward and share our story, we are beginning to realize we have more in common with one another. And when we show our scars to the world we're actually showing people who have also suffered in silence that they no longer have to suffer. When someone shares their scars with me, it makes me feel comfortable to share my scars with them. It opens the dialogue and allows the demons of guilt and shame to fade away.

It's one of the reasons why I took the risk of sharing my story in this book. Because I know how lonely it is to suffer in silence. I have so much to offer my future place of employment because I'm able to draw upon life experiences that are empathetic to people who are suffering. I want to share my message with the world. Your past does not define who are now, or who you will become in the future. Forgiveness exists in our world as the greatest healing force God ever created. It allows us to pick ourselves up and pick a new, brighter future.

DEFINITIⴰN ⴰF SUCCESS

It has not been an easy journey of recovery especially being a journalist in today's toxic climate. I have had to reevaluate my life many times. One of things I have thought a lot about is my definition of success. Is it about fame? Money? Notoriety?

I decided that what was most important to me, and my true measure of success, was helping create a positive impact in people's lives. I want to get my message out into the world about recovery in order to help others in their battle with their own demons. I get great joy hearing people's stories and comments about how something I said helped them in turning their lives around.

My story has been a difficult one to share. In fact, I have had to double my therapy appointments to cope, as I have had to go through my personal traumas again to be able to put them in print. It has been an echo of a cage I once kept closed and locked against my heart. Even though I have opened the cage and it no longer exists, I still feel the soreness and the scars it left within me.

KEEPING POSITIVE

I was warned before I ever jumped in front of the camera that I had better have thick skin because viewers can be ruthless:

"I hate that color tie."

"Seriously, why do you wear eyeliner?"

"Take your gay ass to another state. We don't want your kind here!"

When I am on the air, I get between 50 to 200 messages a day from viewers. Nine out of ten are very positive comments. Why is it that we always focus on the one negative comment? Since when did 10% become greater than 90%? Now, admittedly, I sucked at math in school. But I still know that 90 is way bigger than 10. I also know that anyone would love to have a 90% approval rating.

But still, so many of us focus on the negative. Have you logged onto social media lately? I used to have a Twitter account with a decent following. When I moved to Arizona in 2013, I realized I had moved to an extremely conservative state. It didn't take long for the Twitter wars to start. Our country is really in a messed-up state when a journalist fact-checks the president for one of his thousands of lies, and yet his die-hard followers still refuse to believe the truth. I'm not talking about all Trump supporters. I know quite a few people at my tennis club who voted for him. These are powerful CEOs who will admit they either chose Trump to grow their own bank account, or they voted for him simply because they could not stand Hillary Clinton. Then there are the die-hard peeps referred to as Trump's base. These people will support the president even if, as he said, "I could walk down 5th Avenue and shoot someone and they would still vote for me." I mean, seriously, we have a president who just talked about how he could murder someone in broad daylight and his fans cheer.

I will never forget when my news station sent me to Las Vegas in December 2015 to cover one of the first presidential debates. It was a circus. Sixteen candidates on stage insulting each other with such vehement pettiness. Talking about hand size (referring to

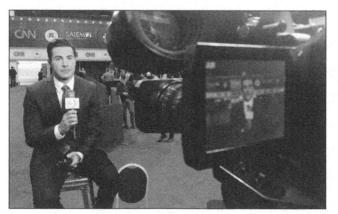

Me covering the 2016 Republican Presidential Debate in Las Vegas

penis size—gross). Watching it in person was even more puzzling. These were people who were supposed to appeal to our best selves. Yet we witnessed several candidates jump into a pit and sling mud at each other.

Sadly, that wasn't the most alarming thing I witnessed. We, the media, were verbally assaulted at every stop on the campaign trail. I even saw a guy wearing a shirt that read "Rope. Tree. Journalist. Some assembly required." That's not freedom of speech. That's

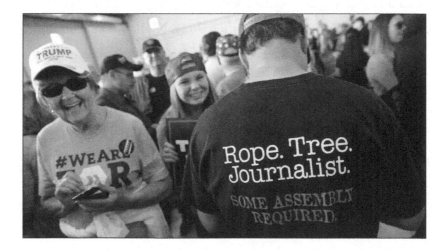

hate speech, and it's threatening. Every single time Trump steps in front of a microphone he throws red meat to his supporters by trashing the media, calling us scum, trash, liars, fake, and "enemy of the people." When the president of the country calls reporters the enemy he is giving cover to his supporters to spew hate and cause harm.

Here's how I responded to viewers who emailed me telling me that I am part of the fake news media and I am the enemy for not supporting Trump. First off, my job as a journalist is NOT to support the president. The late-night Fox News cable hosts do enough cheerleading for him. They are hosts. Entertainers. They are not journalists. They don't have sources. Wait, yes they do. Their source is Trump. Someone who has told thousands of lies in less than two years in office. Trump calls the Fox hosts Hannity, Laura Ingraham, and Rush Limbaugh and tells them whatever it is he wants them to say. And they do it. Nightly. They are doing the president's bidding. But because they lavish praise on the president, he doesn't criticize them.

I would tell his die-hard supporters that it's my job to report the truth. It is my job to fact-check the president. That's the role of the media. Just because the facts don't align with your beliefs doesn't make it fake news.

I want everyone reading this to understand that the media plays a vital role to democracy. The media holds the powerful accountable. We hold politicians' feet to the fire to make sure they aren't wasting taxpayer money. Without the media, you wouldn't know how corrupt some politicians can be. Even with the hate, bigotry, and ignorance that backs our current political environment, it is important to stay positive and strong.

When I came to Arizona in 2013, I wasn't sure what to expect. As an anchor, you don't know how a new audience will react to you. Will they like you? Will they watch? It's a risk we take when we move to a new city. I didn't know anyone in Arizona. I had to start over, and as much as I enjoy a good adventure, it was the first time in my life that I wasn't excited about starting all over again.

At times, living in Arizona was hard for me. It was hard for me to make friends. I went on one date in the five years I lived there. But Arizona turned out to be a huge blessing in my life. For the first time, I had to look inward. I was so alone that I had no one else to focus on but me. It's the reason I finally chose to see a shrink. That decision was the best decision I have ever made, aside from choosing to get sober.

I began meeting my therapist two to three times a month. We worked through some serious issues already talked about in this book: childhood rape, drug abuse, the rest. It took years to work through these issues. But doing so stripped me of all the fakery and narcissistic traits I had layered on top of my true self.

I am very good at reading people. I don't have book smarts. I have street smarts. It's one of the traits that has made me a good reporter. I could go into the ghetto and get gang members to talk to me. But it also has negative side effects. I would often figure out what someone wanted and I would become that. I would become what you wanted me to be rather than just be my authentic self. A few years of sitting on a comfy couch with my shrink changed my perspective and my life. It didn't happen overnight, but I started to peel back the layers of fakery and by doing so revealed my true self.

For the first time in my life, at age 36, I was living my authentic life. I was no longer afraid or ashamed to tell people about my dark past.

When the controversy about Alabama senate candidate Roy Moore came out, I decided it was time to tell my story and speak my truth for the first time publicly. I did the same thing about my past struggles with drug abuse. The opioid crisis was all over the news. I even did a documentary about the heroin/ opioid crisis. Again, I felt compelled to share publicly my own struggles because people kept assuming these drug addicts were scum. Trash. Homeless. Poor. I couldn't let people believe that only "scum" did drugs.

I attempted to put a real face on the crisis, because it was affecting everything from the stay-at-home soccer mom to that guy you watch on the nightly news. The crisis has continued so long and in quiet because people think it is the person begging on the street corner that is the addict, not the woman who is sitting next to you at your children's PTA meeting. It was important to share my struggles because people need to know that addiction does not discriminate. Addiction kills the rich, the poor, the homeless, the upper class, the lower class, black, white, brown; it doesn't matter. Until we accept this truth as a society we will continue to have a drug crisis in this country.

While reading the more than five thousand messages I received when I left Arizona, I had tears streaming down my face. I never knew I had such an impact on people's lives. It wasn't because I read a teleprompter smoothly. It's not because I thrive on covering breaking news. It's not because I'm a political junkie who loves a good debate. These messages were all about me sharing my struggles and sharing with people about how I was able to face them, work through them, and finally reach the light at the end of a dark tunnel. As of this moment, I have been gone from Arizona for about 6 months. I miss it. I hope to get back there someday. Life is funny sometimes.

CANCER IN THE ROOM

It wasn't enough for me to just become sober. I wanted to become the best version of myself. I can tell you, after ten years of sobriety, becoming the best version of myself is not becoming a marble sculpture. When an artist chisels a block of marble and reveals the figure inside, they eventually stop chiseling and begin to smooth and polish their art, and eventually, they walk away and they are finished. Some artists never want to view what they have created again; they just want to move on to the next block.

Creating the best version of ourselves is not something we create and then are done with. It is a work in progress that constantly needs work, rework, and adjustments. People are like sandcastles on a shoreline.

There are parts of my character that I do not like mostly because they are at odds with the person I want to be. Character flaws don't go away, and we have to be alert or they can creep back into our repertoire. As humans, imperfect beings, we often ascribe to the law of entropy in our lives. That is, we seek our lowest, most comfortable level. We act in a way that is familiar to us, and even if we are successful at changing that habit, if we are not careful, we can easily fall back into that habit.

This does not make us a weak person or a bad person. It just makes us human. The good news is that there is a cure that, when administered on a regular basis, can be like a flu shot. That cure is prayer. Handing over our lives to a higher power. Naked. Unadorned. No excuses. Humble and ready for healing.

My point is, changing our lives takes work. Really hard work. And it takes time. Even when we think we are done, some wave comes from nowhere and threatens to level our beautifully built sand castle. What do you do when this happens? You pick up your shovel and start again, but this time, you may do it a little further from the shore. You may build a moat, or you may build the castle even bigger and more sturdy.

My biggest defect of character is that I'm a chameleon. I have this ability to blend into my surroundings. This began as a survival tool when I was a kid. For example, I loved lip synching to Cyndi Lauper and Whitney Houston as a kid. Why? My sisters did it. My sisters would even paint my nails. When it came time to go to school, I couldn't tell anyone about that because I would get teased. We all sort of become chameleons at times in our lives. Like, when I moved to Atlanta. Within months of me being there I was wearing khaki pants and polo shirts, just like a good Southerner. I even ditched hip hop music for country music. I sold my sports car and bought a Ford F-150 truck. When in Rome...

Knowledge is power. And the fact that I am aware of my character defects means I can see negativity from a mile away and I can choose to avoid it or shut it down. I build my sand castle further from the breaking waves.

I've told you about the litmus test I use for every relationship in my life: If you push me closer to my spiritual center, you stay. If you pull me from that spiritual center, you're out of my life. The same can be said for toxic people. We all know them in our lives. No matter what happens, they're always the victim. They make it seem that all this bad stuff is happening to them and it's unfair. These people are the first to want to bring you down into the mud with them, because pigs love company.

One of the ways I have seen this manifest, especially in an office environment, is through gossip. Gossip in any form is toxic. It's gross. It's immature. It's hurtful. We've all been guilty of it and it never leads to anything good. In the TV world, gossip is everywhere and the knives are always cleverly hidden behind people's backs. It's one of those industries where there are probably one thousand people actively trying to figure out how to steal your job. Some of the worst people start rumors or gossip about you thinking that it will ruin your reputation. Others gossip because they're insecure about their own lives and it makes them feel good for a few moments to knock another person down. Know this: gossip will only poison your spirit and your soul and it will NEVER lead to anything good, because the truth always comes out and you will eventually pay the price.

I've been the victim of toxic gossip. There was a rumor flying around West Hollywood, the gay epicenter of America, that I was HIV+. Now, was I promiscuous? Yes. Was a drug addict? Yes. Was a behaving irresponsibly? Absolutely. Am I HIV positive? No. I am not. I know this may seem hypocritical since at one point in my life I was a bug chaser, but the facts is, I have never been HIV+. When I was a bug chaser I was a ticking time bomb, but I was not chasing when this rumor surfaced.

Why would another guy go around telling scores of people that I'm HIV+ when the only person who would know that information is me and my doctor? And since I'm not HIV+, this guy made up a lie and spread it to an entire community. He probably did it out of spite or jealousy. HIV comes with a huge stigma attached to it, unfortunately. I have many friends with HIV and it pains me to see people discriminate against them as if they're damaged goods.

In 2006, I dated a guy from New York City who was HIV+. I was a little scared when he first told me about his status, but then

I educated myself and that fear about contracting the disease went away. I had people ask me, "OMG, how can you date X when you know he's HIV+? Aren't you afraid you'll get infected?" Again, it's none of your business to judge my relationships just as it's none of my business what you think of me.

So how do you avoid gossip? Like I mentioned, gossiping to yourself isn't fun. You need someone to "spill the tea" to or indulge your toxicity. We've all been in situations where a friend calls us up, we go out to lunch, and they begin to rip into one of the friends in your mutual circle. "Did you see Mark last night? I heard he was holding another guy's hands at the bar. He has a boyfriend. That's so shady."

Now, I have two ways I can handle this situation. I can indulge my friend for a little brunch gossip and at the end of brunch feel gross for talking about another friend behind his back, or I can shut it down: "Hey, we weren't there. We don't know if that's true. If you're really concerned, call Mark and ask him. But its none of our business. If we didn't see it, then we shouldn't go around telling people about something we didn't actually see for ourselves. Next topic."

BOOM, the hammer is dropped. When you shut down a toxic person by refusing to indulge their gossipy ways, they will eventually stop coming to you. Because, after all, gossiping is only fun when another person plays along.

DEVELOPING A MORAL COMPASS

In sobriety, people talk all the time about having a spiritual awakening. Addicts who get clean begin to see the miracles, big and small. Some call it their ah-ha moment. Others who prefer more biblical terms refer to it as their burning bush moment. Regardless, if we get clean, stay clean, and commit to a higher power, one day, eventually, God will reveal gifts to us.

I always prided myself for being friends with my exes after we break up. I felt that was a mature quality about me. If the intimate relationship didn't work out, why does that mean we have to completely cut off that relationship. There had to be good reason why I was in the relationship to begin with, right?

MY (RE) BIRTHDAY

It was February 22, 2015. I remember the date because it was a significant one in my sobriety. That day I was celebrating my five years sober anniversary. I was living in Arizona and decided to fly home to LA to attend the church where I went to my very first AA meeting.

Up to this point, I always stayed with my ex, Billy, and his husband. They built a mansion in Hollywood Hills. The place is a palace that sits on the edge of a cliff under the famous Hollywood sign, with a pool that looked like you could swim off the edge and into the city skyline. Billy always has guys over. Some of them were really hot. There was food, music, and yes, drugs. Billy was the first guy I ever fell in love with. He's the guy I met in NYC when I moved there to attend NYU. He had this grip over me. A spell that I could not break.

I told Billy that I was coming to LA that weekend to celebrate five years in recovery. I told him I needed to go to a meeting, and they should come with me and then we could all go to dinner to celebrate.

It was Saturday morning, February 22, 9 am. I landed at Burbank Airport. I got into an Uber and headed to Billy's house. I got a text message from Billy. "Hey, where are you? When do you get in today?"

"Oh. I landed and I'm in an Uber headed your way," I replied.

Billy sent a cryptic message back. "Oh, OK. Just a heads up, we've been partying since last night and there's still some guys over."

I will admit my heart sank, but I tried to convince myself that it was no big deal. My driver dropped me off at the Hollywood Hills mansion. I entered through the security gate. I walked up to the front door and I heard the music and felt the bass thumping, the vibration throughout my body. I knocked a few times. Nothing. I knocked louder. Nothing. Then all of a sudden two guys opened the door, totally naked and high on drugs. Trust me, I know the look well. I used to be a master at it.

One of the guys said, "Damn, you're hot. Come to the backyard. We're all skinny dipping right now."

I should have left. I should have done a 180, called the Uber driver to come get me. But I didn't. I was still holding on to past bonds. I told the guy I wanted to put my stuff in my guest room first and then I'd come outside. I walked upstairs to my guest room. I opened the door to find three guys having an orgy.

I closed the door and took my stuff downstairs. I walked out to the backyard and there were at least ten naked guys frolicking around, high on ecstasy. I saw Billy in the pool and I walked over to greet him. He swam to the side to give me a kiss. He saw the look on my face. He knew that face. After all, we dated for years in our early 20s.

I said, "Hey, I'm going to my AA meeting. I am going to do a couple of things after the meeting, and then are we still on for dinner?"

Billy said, "Yes. We are definitely doing dinner tonight."

I turned around and walked away and that's when another guy screamed, "Hey, come back! Get naked with us!"

I couldn't hold back anymore. "Nah, man. I'm good. I have a really exciting day today. I am celebrating five years sober today! I'm on my way to an AA meeting."

Was it true? Yes. Did I say it in a tone to send a message? You're damn right I did.

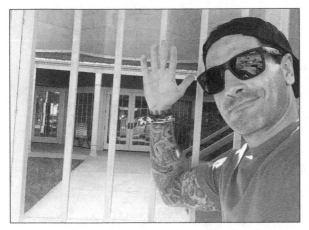

This is the church where I attended my first AA meeting. This is the day I got my 5 year sobriety chip

I left the house and headed to that meeting, the very first place where I admitted I was powerless over drugs and alcohol. I tried to forget the naked orgy that was happening at the house and I focused on being in the moment, at the meeting celebrating something I never thought was possible: five years without picking up a drink or drug.

When they asked, "Is anyone here celebrating an AA birthday?" I raised my hand. I stood up. I said, "Hi, my name is Brandon. I am a grateful RECOVERED addict celebrating five years today!" Everyone clapped. I was so proud of myself.

When I got my five-year chip, I knew exactly what to do with it. I stopped by a flower shop and picked up a beautiful bouquet of white roses. To me they mean spirituality and sympathy and empathy. I got back in my car. I had my five-year chip, the flowers, and a card where I wrote a hand-written message inside.

"Thank you for showing me compassion and love when I was unable and unwilling to love myself. You gave me a second chance at life, and I made a promise to myself that I would make the most out of each day and do my best to spread the message of hope to those who feel helpless as I once did.

"Here's a token of my appreciation. It's my five-year chip. I showed up here on life support. You never gave up on me even though I gave up on myself. You showed me compassion when I showed disdain. You brought me back to life, twice.

"Forever grateful, Brandon L."

I walked into the Hollywood Presbyterian Hospital in Los Angeles. I went to the security guard and said, "Sir. May I go back to the ER to tell the staff thank you?"

He said, "I'm sorry. No. You cannot go back there. I will take those back."

I said, "OK. I understand. Just let them know that they brought me back to life twice in 72 hours. I was on life support after two drug overdoses. I just celebrated five years sober today and wanted to give them my five-year sobriety chip."

The guard looked like he'd seen a ghost. Then a tear rolled down his face. He said, "Oh no, no, no. I'm taking you back there."

We passed the locked doors and headed down a long, narrow

hallway. There were doctors and nurses moving, shouting, saving lives all around me. It was a Saturday, after all, and you can imagine what the ER looks like on a weekend in Los Angeles.

We reached the main area in the ER and the guard tracked down the head ER doctor and brought her over to me. At first, she had an incredulous look on her face. The guard introduced us, and I told her who I was and what happened. Suddenly her face changed. She started to smile. She started to cry. She turned around and whistled loudly. It got everyone's attention.

"I need everyone's attention. Please gather round. This gentleman has something to say."

I was scared, nervous, butterflies in my stomach. Could I say what I needed to? I had to try. I opened my mouth and out came, "I just want to say thank you. I came here five years ago addicted to meth. I had bleeding in my brain. I was in a coma. I gave up. But you kept believing that I could live. You have no clue the impact you've all made on my life. I have made it my life's mission to save as many addicts as I can from death."

I couldn't stop crying. Everyone was bawling. Nurses came to give me a hug. And then, there she was. The nurse who gave me clothes when I was brought to the ER naked. The nurse who gave me the $10 she had in her purse so that I could get home. The nurse who told me about AA. The nurse who told me, "God will always believe in you even when you don't believe in him." She was crying. I was crying. My soul was full of love.

Whenever I have a bad day, I try to remember those beautiful God moments in my recovery to show me that life isn't bad. We may have some bumps in the road, but we have to keep our eyes open to the miracles. They happen when we do things selflessly for others.

As I drove to the Hollywood Hills mansion, I had an epiphany. I pulled to the side of the road before pulling into the driveway. I sat there quietly. It all made sense. I started to smile. God was showing me a very important life lesson. God was showing and telling me this: "Brandon, this morning you saw what your old life looked like. Sex. Drugs. Orgies. I also showed you what your life is like today. Spiritual. Loving. Caring. Sober."

Wow. What a beautiful message to receive on such an important milestone. I walked into the mansion. I grabbed my stuff and left. I was done. The guys called me to ask where I was going. I didn't respond. I didn't know what to say. I wanted to think about it. I just knew I couldn't stay there.

About two weeks went by, and I decided it was time to officially end the friendship. These guys had been such an integral part of my life for decades. This was not going to be easy. I didn't hate them. I wasn't mad at them. I was disappointed. But really, how disappointed could I be when my friends behaved as they always have? It was I who'd changed.

It's been about five years and it's sad sometimes looking back. When you break up with friends, it's like mourning the loss of a loved one. But this needed to be done. I love this saying because it sums it all up for me: *"Just so we're all clear, it's OK to miss people you no longer want in your life."*

HAVE FAITH

The thing I noticed when walking into my first AA meeting was one three-letter word, and it scared the living shit out of me. So much so that I turned around and tried to leave before a few guys came running after me, encouraging me to come back into the meeting. The word that frightened me: God. It was everywhere. It's in the Big Book, which is the AA bible, essentially, and it was in quotes all over the room.

I grew up Catholic. I was confirmed. I went to church school. My parents were not religious, but for some reason they forced me to go to church. Maybe it made them feel like that was good parenting. I'm really not sure why they sent me there other than to conform to societal norms. I never liked it. Probably because I knew down deep that I was a gay kid, and back in the 80s and 90s the Catholic Church railed against homosexuality as sinful. As I previously mentioned, I was told repeatedly gay people who have gay sex will burn in hell. I always found this example to be the most egregious: A priest can be gay, he just can't act out sexually. Wait a second. What kind of rule or exception is that? I can be into another guy and attracted to him, but God forbid I get naked with that man.

Anti-gay groups to this day believe that gay marriage will be what ends America. Excuse me while I spit out my coffee from laughing. When in doubt, just blame the gays for the destruction of marriage. Right. I should point out that the divorce rate is already above 50% from straight couples, yet these same anti-gay pro-family groups have no problem with straight men divorcing multiple times and remarrying umpteen times. Nope. Nothing to see here. Pick and choose whichever Bible verse fits your argument.

When I walked into that AA room, those feelings of being ridiculed came roaring back. Those suppressed feelings as a child came rising to the surface. When my first sponsor asked me, "Brandon, how is your relationship with God?" I quipped, "I don't have one."

"That's OK, Brandon. I don't want you to focus on the word God right now. We will come back to that later." We continued doing our step work.

One of the suggestions my sponsor gave me was to meditate. Honestly, even meditating made me uncomfortable. The thought of being silent and sitting there was just weird to me. About 45 seconds into meditating I start thinking about what I'm going to make for dinner or what meetings I have to plan for. But I followed his suggestion about prayer.

He asked me, "Brandon, do you pray?"

"I told you I don't have a relationship with God, so why would I pray?" I replied.

"That's OK. I want you to do it anyway. When you wake up every morning and when you go to bed each night, I want you to get open your knees and pray," he said.

"So, you want me to pray to a God I don't believe in?"

He smiled and replied, "That's exactly what I want you to do."

I did commit at our first meeting that I was open and willing to do whatever was needed to get and stay sober. So, I started praying. I will admit, it was really weird at first. Do I talk out loud? Do I whisper?

Over the course of the six months we were doing step work, I wrote about all my near-death experiences. I shared about the two times in one week I ended up in the same ER on life support. I shared about getting high while skiing and going off a cliff, landing on my neck and thinking I was paralyzed. I reflected on falling asleep on the 110 freeway in downtown LA and waking up at 4 am in the emergency lane with my hazards on and my seat fully reclined.

"Don't you believe now? Don't you believe something was keeping you alive? You should be dead ten times over. But you're not. You're right here. Alive. Talking with me about how you are a SURVIVOR!" my sponsor said.

You notice how he never mentioned that three little word, GOD? He stopped mentioning that around me. Instead, he phrased it differently. He asked me, "Don't you see now that something greater than you was keeping you around?"

Finally, my sponsor opened the door to believing in something I like to call a higher power. You've heard me say that repeatedly, *higher power.*

"Brandon, you don't have to believe in God to get sober. You don't have to believe in God. Period."

"I don't?"

"Nope. You don't. But let me ask you this. After reflecting on all your near-death experiences, do you believe that something saved you? Something was protecting you?"

I thought to myself: well, hell. I don't think I'm that lucky to be alive. I had too many near-death experiences to even try to explain how luck was always on my side. That made no sense. I finally admitted something I never thought would come out of this addict's mouth: something greater than me was real, and it saved me from death.

"Do you believe in anything greater or more powerful than you?" my sponsor asked.

I was still early in recovery and had a larger-than-life ego. There were times I was on drugs when I felt truly invincible. I felt like Superman. But, the reality was staring me in the face. It was written down on medical records. All the times I should have been dead, something greater than me was keeping me around. Miracles had occurred in my life, but I had been too self-absorbed to see them.

"I do," I replied. "I do believe something—I don't know what it is—but something is protecting me."

Over time, this feeling has become more powerful. The longer I'm sober, the stronger that bond with my higher power is. I pray every single night and every single morning. I can't fall asleep until I do. My sponsor was having me act the part by praying, knowing that one day that action would lead to belief. And it did. Growth is uncomfortable. It's awkward. It's scary. My higher power can't be seen. I can feel it. When I pray that my higher power remove my defects of character (which is often my ego) I am more present to my higher power.

Having faith is so much better than not having it at all. I have relied on my spirituality and my spiritual connection with my higher power so many times in sobriety. Whether it's losing a job or dealing with family, having faith allows to me to turn my will over to my higher power. I believe so much in my higher power that I rarely stress about my job, my income, my finances or relationships. I truly believe that my higher power will take care of me. I have no reason to believe that it won't.

I say this to non-believers: Life is easier when you can rely on faith than nothing at all. What do you have to lose to give it a try?

For me, it took the physical exercise of writing down on paper all the near-death experiences. Then, I wrote down how many incredible people came into my life once I was sober and compared those friendships to the friends I had when I was using. The differences were striking. My higher power was giving me everything I needed at just the right time. Incredible people have come into my life and I know that it's not luck.

Building a relationship with my higher power is a continuous one. It's only grown stronger the more I commit to it. And why would I stop now? That would be as bad as someone who's depressed who decides to stop taking their medicine because they feel better. If you stop taking that medicine, you will just revert to the same negative thoughts and behaviors. If spirituality is medicine, then sign me up for automatic refills. I'd much rather overdose on spirituality than pills. Just sayin'.

So many of us search for the answer to the question: "What is God's will for me?" The answer for me is: to help others who are struggling just as others showed me there was a better way to live. The people I met at my first AA meeting gave me hope. My sole purpose is pass that hope onto others. I can't save the world. None of us can. But we have the ability to share our experience, strength, and hope to impact others' lives.

Made in the USA
Las Vegas, NV
04 April 2021